WORK-RELATED MUSCULOSKELETAL DISORDERS DUE TO COMPUTER USE

Orhan KORHAN

WORK-RELATED MUSCULOSKELETAL DISORDERS DUE TO COMPUTER USE

A Literature Review

LAP LAMBERT Academic Publishing

Impressum/Imprint (nur für Deutschland/ only for Germany)
Bibliografische Information der Deutschen Nationalbibliothek: Die Deutsche Nationalbibliothek verzeichnet diese Publikation in der Deutschen Nationalbibliografie; detaillierte bibliografische Daten sind im Internet über http://dnb.d-nb.de abrufbar.

Coverbild: www.ingimage.com

Verlag: LAP LAMBERT Academic Publishing AG & Co. KG
Dudweiler Landstr. 99, 66123 Saarbrücken, Deutschland
Telefon +49 681 3720-310, Telefax +49 681 3720-3109
Email: info@lap-publishing.com

Herstellung in Deutschland:
Schaltungsdienst Lange o.H.G., Berlin
Books on Demand GmbH, Norderstedt
Reha GmbH, Saarbrücken
Amazon Distribution GmbH, Leipzig
ISBN: 978-3-8383-6625-8

Imprint (only for USA, GB)
Bibliographic information published by the Deutsche Nationalbibliothek: The Deutsche Nationalbibliothek lists this publication in the Deutsche Nationalbibliografie; detailed bibliographic data are available in the Internet at http://dnb.d-nb.de.

Cover image: www.ingimage.com

Publisher: LAP LAMBERT Academic Publishing AG & Co. KG
Dudweiler Landstr. 99, 66123 Saarbrücken, Germany
Phone +49 681 3720-310, Fax +49 681 3720-3109
Email: info@lap-publishing.com

Printed in the U.S.A.
Printed in the U.K. by (see last page)
ISBN: 978-3-8383-6625-8

TABLE OF CONTENTS

SECTION PAGE

1. The Significance of the Study..3

2. Work-Related Musculoskeletal Disorders (WRMSDs)..4

3. Signs and Symptoms of Musculoskeletal Disorders..7

4. Types of Musculoskeletal Disorders...8

5. The Nature of WRMSDs...10

6. Economic Impact and Lost Productivity...12

7. Computers and WRMSDs...13

8. Postures..29

9. Psychosocial Factors...37

10. Physical Factors...43

11. Psychological Factors...47

12. Effect of Interventions...48

References...53

THE NATURE OF WORK-RELATED MUSCULOSKELETAL DISORDERS DUE TO COMPUTER USE

1. The Significance of the Study

The National Institute for Occupational Safety and Health (NIOSH) in the USA defines a Musculoskeletal Disorder (MSD) as a disorder that affects a part of the body's musculoskeletal system, which includes bones, nerves, tendons, ligaments, joints, cartilage, blood vessels and spinal discs. These are the injuries that result from repeated motions, vibrations and forces placed on human bodies while performing various job actions. The factors that can contribute to musculoskeletal symptoms include heredity, physical condition, previous injury, pregnancy, poor diet, and lifestyle.

Work-related musculoskeletal symptoms occur when there is a mismatch between the physical requirements of the job and the physical capacity of the human body. Musculoskeletal disorders are work-related when the work activities and work conditions significantly contribute to their development, but not necessarily the sole or significant determinant of causation. Work-related musculoskeletal disorders (WRMSDs) describe a wide range of inflammatory and degenerative conditions affecting the muscles, tendons, ligaments, joint, peripheral nerves, and supporting blood vessels. These conditions result in pain and functional impairment and may affect neck, shoulders, elbows, forearms, wrists and hands.

The causes of musculoskeletal disorders in the workplace are diverse and poorly understood. The meaning that working has to an individual may help to explain why certain psychological factors are associated with musculoskeletal discomfort and may eventually provide one way to intervene to reduce MSD.

Musculoskeletal disorders have been observed and experienced widely at workplaces where the computers are frequently used. Increase in the number of employees working with computer and mouse coincides with an increase of work-related musculoskeletal disorders (WRMSDs) and sick leave, which affects the physical health of workers and pose financial burdens on the companies, governmental and non-governmental organizations.

This literature review study begins with the description of the risk factors and types of musculoskeletal disorders, and followed by the discussion of general characteristics of the musculoskeletal disorders. The economic impact of work-related musculoskeletal disorders was reviewed. This was followed by the discussion of issues related with workplace ergonomics, and an extensive review of computer use related upper extremities musculoskeletal disorders. Finally, the literature review is concluded with a discussion of computer keyboarding with different postures and different keyboard designs.

2. Work-Related Musculoskeletal Disorders (WRMSDs)

Orthopedic Clinics of North America (1996) cited the causes of work-related musculoskeletal symptoms in two categories:

A. *Psychosocial factors.* These include monotonous work, time pressure, a high workload, unorganized work-rest schedules, complexity of tasks, career concerns, lack of peer support, a poor relationship between workers and their supervisors, and poor organizational characteristics (climate, culture and communications).

> "Psychosocial factors at work are the subjective aspects as perceived by workers and the managers. They often have the same names as the work organization factors, but are different in that they carry 'emotional' value for the worker. Thus, the nature of the supervision can have positive or negative psychosocial effects (emotional stress), while the work organization aspects are just descriptive of how the supervision is accomplished and do not carry emotional value. Psychosocial factors are the individual subjective perceptions of the work organization factors". (Hagberg 1995)

Organization of work refers to the way work processes are structured and managed. In general, work organization refers to the way work processes are structured and managed, and it deals with subjects such as the following:

- Scheduling of work (work-rest schedules, hours of work and shift work)

- Job design (complexity of tasks, skill and effort required, and the degree of control of work)
- Interpersonal aspects of work (relationships with supervisors and friends)
- Career concerns (job security and growth opportunities)
- Management style (participatory management and teamwork)
- Organizational characteristics (climate, culture and communications).

Many of these elements are referred as "psychosocial factors" and have been recognized as risk factors for job stress and psychological strain. Stress is considered as human body's physical and emotional reaction to circumstances or events that cause frightening, irritation, confusion, danger or excitement. Particularly, stress is a change from a person's normal behavior in response to something that causes wear and tear on the body's physical or mental resources.

There are internal or external stimuli that cause stress. The internal stimuli are those stressors that involve self-expectations, impersonal barriers and conflicting desires. Apparently, internal stimuli depend on personal aspects. However, external stimuli include situations where expectations, time limit, lack of resources, and lack of vision and goals present.

Stressors may be physiological, psychological, social, environmental, developmental, spiritual or cultural and represents an unmet need. Stress causes changes in the human body that are usually centered on the nervous system and endocrine system. Therefore, human body's internal environment is constantly changing and the body's adaptive mechanisms continually function to adjustments in heart rate, respiratory rate, blood pressure, temperature, fluid and electrolyte balances, hormone secretions and level of consciousness.

It is the extensive and intensive stress that causes the disorders in the musculoskeletal system. The causes of the stress arise due to experience the feelings like frustration, anger, irritation, confusion, nervousness, or tension. Not only the frequency of exposure to these emotions, but also the repetition of the motions and activities cause the musculoskeletal disorders or injuries.

In considering human emotions and feelings, and applying the results of the research to their impact on the musculoskeletal system, it is probably platitudinous to make a statement that the greater the knowledge and understanding of the human being, the better the result obtained. In order to identify and understand the effect of the emotions on the musculoskeletal system, important risk factors for musculoskeletal disorders should be recognized.

B. *Physical factors.* These include intense, repeated, or sustained exertions; awkward, non-neutral, and extreme postures; rapid work pace; repeated and/or prolonged activity; insufficient time for recovery, vibration, and cold temperatures.

1) Awkward postures:

Body postures determine which joints and muscles are used in an activity and the amount of force or stresses that are generated or tolerated. For example, more stress is placed on the spinal discs when lifting, lowering, or handling objects with the back bent or twisted, compared with when the back is straight. Manipulative or other tasks requiring repeated or sustained bending or twisting of the wrists, knees, hips, or shoulders also impose increased stresses on these joints. Activities requiring frequent or prolonged work on wrists and finders, such as keyboarding, can be particularly stressful.

2) Repetitive motions:

If motions are repeated frequently (e.g., every few seconds) and for prolonged periods such as an 8-hour shift, fatigue and muscle-tendon strain can accumulate. Tendons and muscles can often recover from the effects of stretching or forceful exertions if sufficient time is allotted between exertions. Effects of repetitive motions from performing the same work activities are increased when awkward postures and forceful exertions are involved. Repetitive actions as a risk factor can also depend on the body area and specific act being performed.

3) Duration:

Duration refers to the amount of time a person is continually exposed to a risk factor. Job tasks that require use of the same muscles or motions for long durations, such as prolonged typing, increase the likelihood of both localized and general fatigue. In general, the longer the period of continuous work (e.g., tasks requiring sustained muscle contraction), the longer the recovery or rest time required.

4) Frequency:

Frequency refers to how many times a person repeats a given exertion within a given period of time. Of course, the more often the exertion is repeated, the greater the speed of movement of the body part being exerted. Also, recovery time decreases the more frequently an exertion is completed. And, as with duration, this increases the likelihood of both localized and general fatigue.

C. ***Psychological Risk Factors***

In addition to the above conditions, other aspects of work may not only contribute to physical stress but psychological stress as well. While the human body is, indeed, a mechanism limited in motions by virtue of the biological characteristics of the body, it also contains a thinking, reasoning, feeling brain. Human beings experience pain, joy, sadness, depression, anger, boredom, frustration, fear, outrage, jealousy, love hate, and (even) schizophrenia.

Responses such as anxiety, tension, depression, anger, frustration, fear, fatigue, confusion, helplessness, and lack of vigor arise when the human being exposed to stress.

3. Signs and Symptoms of Musculoskeletal Disorders

(a) A decreased range of motion, such as restricted or limited movement, and pain in the joints (knee, elbow, wrist, neck, or shoulder),
(b) Abnormal formation of extremities, such as curled fingers or toes,
(c) A noticeable decrease in grip strength, making it difficult to hold and lift objects,

(d) A loss of muscle function or control, which can cause feeling of heaviness or clumsiness in the affected area,

(e) Fingers or toes turning white,

(f) Muscles in the forearm become irritated and soft tissues become inflamed and swollen and press on the nearby nerves and cause neurophysiological changes,

(g) Sensations such as pain, numbness, tingling, burning, cramping of stiffness. (Occupational Safety and Health Administration, 1999)

4. Types of Musculoskeletal Disorders

1. Tendonitis: It is the most common hand problem, which happens when the tendons connecting the fingers to muscles in the forearms get inflamed. Tendons help attach muscle to bone to allow movement of a joint (OSHA, 1999).

2. Tenosynovitis: This is another common ailment, where fluid-filled sacks (synovial sheaths) that surround and protect the tendons swell. This swelling can also lead to a condition known as Carpal Tunnel Syndrome. The carpal tunnel, a small opening near the bottom of the hand, is just big enough to house the tendons and the median nerve, which provides sensation to the hand. When the synovial sheaths swell the carpal tunnel becomes cramped, putting pressure on the nerve. The symptoms of carpal tunnel syndrome vary, but often include numbness, tingling or a burning sensation in the palms, fingers and wrists. Over time, the condition can lead to loss of strength and sensation in the hand (OSHA, 1999).

3. Nerve Compression: Nerves that transmit signals from body parts to the brain are located throughout the body. They often run through small tunnels and between vertebrae in the spine. Various conditions can cause nerves to become squeezed, pinched or compressed. This can result in shooting pain, numbness, weakness and loss of coordination. Sciatica occurs when the sciatic nerve in the spine become compressed. Symptoms appear in the back of the leg and side of the foot. Carpal Tunnel Syndrome also occurs when swelling causes the median nerve in the wrist to become compressed (OSHA, 1999).

4. Raynaud's Syndrome/Disease: This is a loss of blood circulation, which results in whitening and numbness of the finders. It is sometimes called "white finger", "wax finger" or "dead finger" (OSHA, 1999).

5. Reflex Sympathetic Dystrophy: This is a rare, incurable condition characterized by fry, swollen hands and loss of muscle control. It is consistently painful (OSHA, 1999).

6. Ganglion Cyst: This disorder arise when a swelling or lump in the wrist resulting from jelly-like substance leaks from a joint or tendon sheath (OSHA, 1999).

7. Cervical Radiculopathy: This is the condition where, an injury at the vertebrae or disks in the neck (cervical vertebrae) could result in pain, numbness or weakness in the shoulder, arm, wrist or hand due to the nerves that extend out from between the cervical vertebrae provide sensation and trigger movement in these areas (OSHA, 1999).

8. Lateral Epicondylitis: This is a condition when the outer part of the elbow becomes painful and tender, usually as a result of a specific strain, overuse, or a direct bang. (OSHA, 1999)

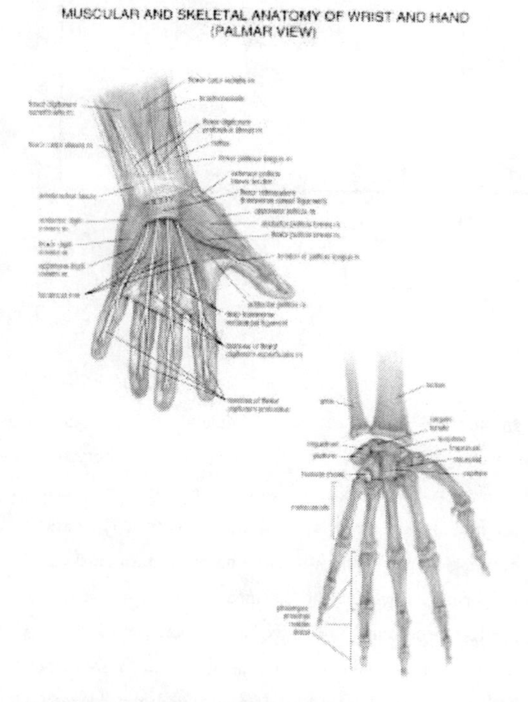

Figure 1. Muscular and Skeletal Anatomy of Wrist and Hand

5. The Nature of WRMSDs

The World Health Organization recognize the conditions that result in pain and functional impairment that affect neck, shoulders, elbows, forearms, wrists, and hands are work-related when the work activities and work conditions significantly contribute to the development of work-related disorders but not as the sole determinant of causation.

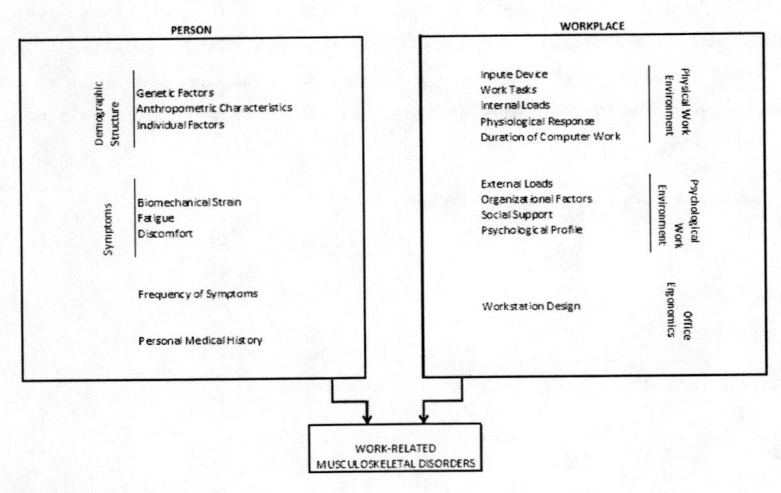

Figure 2. Factors scheme

Baker et al. (2002) thought that the causes of musculoskeletal disorders in the workplace are diverse and poorly understood. Therefore, they conducted an exploratory study to see if there was an association between the meaning of working and musculoskeletal discomfort and if that association was predictive of the severity of the discomfort. They asked 170 to fill out a survey about the meaning of work, and a questionnaire on musculoskeletal discomfort. They entered seven component composites of the meaning of working (work centrality, obligation, entitlement, comfort, promotion/power, expressive, and social support) into a linear multiple regression model. The results suggested that there was a moderate, significant association between overall musculoskeletal discomfort and promotion/power as well as the control variables age, gender, job satisfaction, average hours worked, and site. A logistic linear regression found that these composites, along with social support, could accurately identify who was in a none/mild discomfort category or a moderate/severe discomfort category 72% of the time. The overall pattern suggested that females who worked longer hours, valued promotion and power and disliked social support were most likely to develop moderate to severe musculoskeletal discomfort. Their study provided a preliminary exploration of the association between meaning and musculoskeletal disorders (MSDs) in the workplace.

In their review paper, Aptel et al. (2002) stated that biomechanical factors such as repetitive motion, strenuous efforts, extreme joint postures and/or psychosocial factors establishes the key role work-related musculoskeletal disorders.

Punnet and Wegman (2004) indicated that work-related musculoskeletal disorders are highly prevalent in manual intensive occupations such as clerical work, mainly on upper extremities. They listed the job features that cite as risk factors for musculoskeletal disorders as; rapid work pace, repetitive motion patterns, insufficient recovery time, heavy lifting and forceful manual exertions, non-neutral body postures, pressure concentrations, segmental or whole body vibration, and local or whole body exposure to cold. According to them; age, gender, socio-economic status, ethnicity, obesity, smoking, muscle strength and work capacity are psychosocial risk factors).

McBeth and Jones (2007) examined the rate of musculoskeletal pain in adolescent and adult populations, with a focus on three commonly reported pain disorders: shoulder pain, low back pain and fibromyalgia/chronic widespread pain. Their results showed that there was a paucity of data on musculoskeletal pain in adolescent populations, pain was common, although the actual rates were unclear. Pain was commonly reported among adult populations, with almost one fifth reporting widespread pain, one third shoulder pain, and up to one half reporting low back pain in a 1-month period. They stated that the prevalence of pain varies within specific population subgroups; group factors (including socioeconomic status, ethnicity and race) and individual factors (smoking, diet, and psychological status) were all associated with the reporting of musculoskeletal pain.

Musculoskeletal conditions (MSC) are common throughout the world and their impact on individuals is diverse and manifold. Knowledge of the determinants for disability and of strategies for prevention and rehabilitation management according to the scientific evidence is critical for reducing the burden of MSC. Weigl et al. (2007) reviewed the evidence for common determinants of functioning and disability in patients with MSC. They focused on environmental factors (EF) and personal factors (PF) and have structured them according to the International Classification of Functioning, Disability and Health (ICF) framework. They also discussed prevention strategies, prevention needs to address those EF and PF. Furthermore they described modern principles of rehabilitation and reviewed the evidence for specific rehabilitation interventions.

6. Economic Impact and Lost Productivity

Musculoskeletal disorders of the low back and upper extremities are an important and costly health problem. Apparently this is an important and costly health problem. Musculoskeletal disorders account for nearly 70 million physician office visits in the US annually and an estimated 130 million total health care encounters including outpatient, hospital, and emergency room visits. In 1999, nearly 1 million people took time away from work to treat and recover from work-related musculoskeletal pain. Conservative estimates of the economic burden imposed, as measure by compensation costs, lost wages and lost productivity are between $45-54 billion annually (US Commission on Behavioral and Social Sciences and Education, 2000).

In a national household survey across Great Britain in 1995 estimated that 5.4 million working days are lost annually due to time off work because of work-related neck and upper limb musculoskeletal disorders. That makes approximately 1 month's work is lost annually for each individual case in the UK. The Health and Safety Executive (HSE) in Britain estimated that work-related upper limb disorders incurred an approximate cost of £1.25 billion per year.

In Norway, 15% of all reports are considered to be work-related, 40% in Denmark and Finland, and 70% in Sweden (Broberg, 1996). In Italy, 60% of claims for upper limb musculoskeletal disorders were recognized as occupational diseases and so resulted in compensation.

In France, the percentage of recognized and compensated musculoskeletal disorders compared to total number of occupational ill-health diseases steadily increased from 40% (2602 cases) in 1992 to 63% (5856 cases) in the year 1996 (Helliwell, 1996). Aptel et al.

(2002) stated that work-related musculoskeletal disorders of the upper limb accounted for over two-thirds of all occupational disorders recognized in France. Moreover, in France the cost of low back pain was estimated at nearly 1.3 billion Euros in 1990 (Aptel et al., 2002).

It is believed that direct costs due to compensated work-related musculoskeletal disorders are only a relatively low proportion (30-50%) of the total costs (Hagberg et al., 1995). Borghouts et al. (1999) estimated that the direct cost of neck pain in the Netherlands for 1996 was $160 million and the indirect cost was $527 million, where the direct cost was approximately 30% of the indirect cost.

Toomingas (1998) estimated that about 20-25% of all expenditure for medical care, sick leave and sickness pensions in the Nordic countries in 1991 were related to conditions of the musculoskeletal system (of which 20-80% were work-related). In Sweden, musculoskeletal conditions constituted 15% of all sick-leave days and 18% of all sickness pensions in 1994 (Statistics Sweden, 1997).

Among work related upper extremity disorders, Carpal Tunnel Syndrome (CTS) has the biggest impact in the professional computer users' health and in the industrial related medical and non-medical costs (Fagarasanu and Kumar, 2003). CTS affect over 8 million Americans (U.S. Department of Labor, 1999). From the 37,804 cases of work-related CTS reported in 1994, 7897 (21%) were attributed to repetitive typing or key entry data (Szabo, 1998). In the U.S. alone, approximately 260,000 carpal tunnel release operations are performed each year, with 47% of the cases considered to be work related. Almost half of the carpal tunnel cases resulted in 31 days or more of work loss (U.S. National Center for Health Statistics, 2000). The non-medical costs of a CTS case from compensation settlement and disability average $10,000/hand. This sum is increased by the medical cost and indirect costs that raises it to $20,000-$100,000/hand (Szabo, 1998). Up to 36% of all CTS patients require lifelong medical treatment (U.S. Department of Labor, 1999).

7. Computers and WRMSDs

In 1984, only 25 percent of the population used computers every day in their jobs. By 1993, that number had climbed considerably to an estimated 45 percent and has continued to climb ever since. The Occupational Safety and Health Administration estimates that over 18 million workers must perform extensive keyboarding as part of their jobs.

Later in 1996, more than 647,000 American workers experienced serious injuries due to overexertion or repetitive motion on the job. These work-related musculoskeletal disorders (WMSDs) account for 34 percent of lost workday injuries. WMSDs cost employers an estimated $15 to $20 billion in workers' compensation costs in 1995 and $45 to $60 billion more in indirect costs. ("Occupational Safety and Health Administration", Feb 1999)

The US Census Bureau reported that, in the USA (1999), half of employed adults used a computer in their jobs and the trend still continues (http://www.census.gov/population/pop-profile/1999/chap10.pdf). It has been reported that 27% of office workers who work with a computer have discomfort in the neck and shoulder (Sauter et al., 1991).

More than half of the working population (both males and females) in the European Community use computers in their daily work. Increased computer use time for work purposes tends to an increased incidence of work-related musculoskeletal disorders among computer users. High prevalence of health disturbances has been associated with constrained posture, poor ergonomics design of the work place, input devices as well as of stress related factors (Editorial, 2002).

Intensive computer use is associated with an increased risk of neck, shoulder, elbow, wrist and hand pain, paresthesias and numbness. Repetition, forceful exertions, awkward positions and localized contact stress are associated with the development of upper limb cumulative trauma in computer users. The repetitive computer use such as typing the keyboard and drig-drag the mouse overload neck, shoulder, arm and hand muscles and joints. As they continue to be overworked cumulative trauma happens (Ming and Zaproudina 2003).

Carpal tunnel syndrome (CTS) is the most commonly reported work-related musculoskeletal disorder of the upper extremity. Matias et al. (1998) worked on a study to develop a theoretically based operational quantitative predictive model of the risk of work-related carpal tunnel syndrome (CTS) among VDT (video display terminal) operators. They collected data on job exposure, anthropometry and posture factors using questionnaires, direct observation and video-recordings. In order to develop operational models, they performed discriminant analysis and logistic regression. They found out that percentage of workday working with a VDT was the most significant factor and accounted for 60% of the variance explaining the causation of musculoskeletal discomforts associated with CTS, and using the logistic regression model, increasing the daily work duration from 1 hour to 4 hours increases the probability of CTS risk from 0.45 to 0.92. The results of their study suggested that the main causation of CTS is job design, the secondary is posture associated with the workplace design and the least contributing factor to CTS causation is the individual's anthropometric make-up.

Babski-Reeves and Young (2002) compared the accuracy of measures commonly used to quantify repetition (cycle time (CT), number of hand movements (HM), and exposure classification (EC)) (i.e. high and low repetition), in predicting CTS and positive findings for CTS. Participant exposure to repetition was quantified through direct and video observation of operators within a processing facility. Their logistic regression result indicate that for diagnosed CTS, HM were the only repetition measure to have a significant relationship, and was tentatively concluded to be the best predictor. Three interactions were also found to have significant relationships with diagnosed CTS. No statistically significant results were found for positive findings for CTS.

Jensen et al. (2002) studied associations between duration of computer and mouse use and musculoskeletal symptoms among computer users. They delivered a questionnaire with a 69% participation rate. Logistic regression analyses on full-time working employees showed that working almost the whole working day with a computer was associated with neck symptoms and shoulder symptoms among women and hand symptoms among men. Among respondents working almost all of their work time with a computer the gender and age-adjusted odds ratio for mouse use more than half of the work time was 1.68 for hand/wrist symptoms. Call center and data entry workers experienced the lowest possibilities for development at work.

Blatter and Bonger (2002) examined the association between work-related upper limb disorders (WRULDs) and duration of computer and mouse use, to investigate differences in these associations between men and women, and examined whether a possible relationship between duration of computer use and WRULDs was explained by physical or psychosocial risk factors. Participants had filled out a questionnaire on job characteristics, job content, physical workload, psychosocial workload and musculoskeletal symptoms. Working with a computer during more than 6 h/day was associated with WRULDs in all body regions. Their analyses showed that the strength of the associations differed between men and women. In men, only moderate associations were seen for computer use more than 6 h/day. In women, moderately increases were observed for duration of computer use of more than 4 h/day and strongly increased risks for a computer use during more than 6 h/day.

Amell and Kumar (1999) reviewed the state of the relationship between computer keyboard use and the development of cumulative trauma disorders (CTDs). They also reviewed alternative keyboard designs using biomechanical evaluation methods as justification for their use. They discusses on the critical factors such as repetitiveness of the keyboarding task, the tendency of users to type with excessive force and forcing the users to maintain prolonged awkward and static postures in relation to the CTD development.

Tittiranonda et al. (1999) participated in a randomized, placebo-controlled trial evaluation of the effects of pain severity, functional hand status, and comfort on four different computer keyboards (the apple adjustable keyboard [kb1], comfort keyboard system [kb2], Microsoft natural keyboard [kb3], and placebo) on eighty computer users with musculoskeletal disorders. Compared to placebo, kb3 and to a lesser extent kb1 groups demonstrated an improving trend in pain severity and hand function. However, there was no corresponding consistent improvement in clinical findings in the alternative geometry keyboard groups compared to the placebo group. Overall, there was a significant correlation between improvement of pain and severity and greater satisfaction with the keyboards. Their results provide evidence that keyboard users may experience a reduction in hand pain after several months of use of some alternative geometry keyboards.

Computer pointing devices such as the mouse are widely used. Despite this, the relationship between musculoskeletal symptoms and mouse use has not been established. Cook et al. (2000) conducted a cross-sectional study to determine whether a relationship existed between computer mouse use and musculoskeletal symptoms in a sample of 270 computer mouse users. Factors demonstrating significant associations with symptoms were entered into a step-wise multiple logistic regression. They found no relationship between hours of mouse use per day and reported symptoms. A relationship was found between the variable of arm abduction which is specific to mouse use and symptoms in the neck. Relationships were found between non-mouse specific risk factors such as stress, screen height and shoulder elevation. The findings of their study support the hypothesis that mouse use may contribute to musculoskeletal injury of the neck and upper extremity. Mouse users are exposed to the same recognized risk factors associated with keyboard use as well as the additional risk factor of arm abduction during mouse use.

Harvey and Peper (1997) discussed the applications of sEMG (surface electromyography) for evaluation of alternative computer pointing device use, appropriate ergonomics equipment design, and a methodology for improving muscle awareness, strengthening, relaxation, and work style practices to promote healthier computer use. They examined muscle tension and subjective muscle tension awareness while using a computer mouse positioned to the right of a standard computer keyboard and a centrally positioned trackball. Seventeen volunteer subjects participated in their study and all subject showed significantly higher mean sEMG activity recorded from the upper trapezius, right posterior deltoid, and right lower trapezius/rhomboids during mouse use to the right of a standard keyboard compared to using a trackball positioned centrally ($p<0.001$).

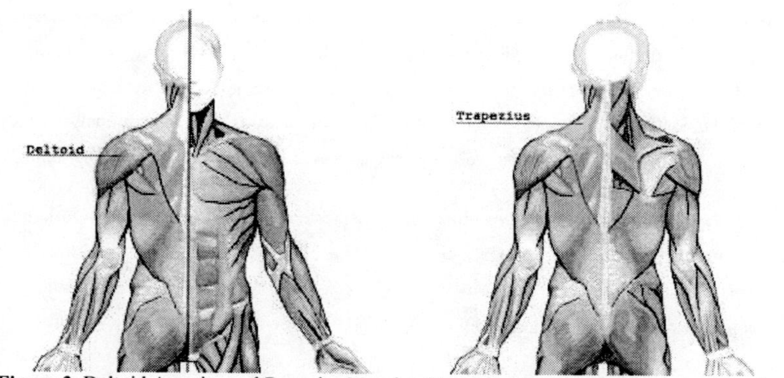

Figure 3. Deltoid Anterior and Posterior Muscles, Trapezius Anterior and Posterior Muscles

Tasks similar to mousing, such as keyboarding, have been shown to result in static muscle loading of the shoulder, therefore the potential may also exist for an increased neck and upper limb disorder with mouse use. Cooper and Straker (1998) indicated that as the computer mouse as an input device is increasing, the studies towards directly addressing the related musculoskeletal problems are not adequate. They compared the dominant shoulder muscle load from upper trapezius and anterior deltoid, postures and discomfort during mousing and keyboarding. In their study, eight subjects performed a 10 minute computer task with both mouse and keyboard input. They collected posture and rating of discomfort EMG readings from anterior deltoid and upper trapezius muscle. The differences in EMG readings showed that increased anterior deltoid loads with mouse use and decreased trapezius loads.

In their review paper, Fagarasanu and Kumar (2003) outlined relevant information about Carpal Tunnel Syndrome (CTS) risk factors present in data entry task and their implications, with a special emphasis on different extreme postures determined by conventional and alternate keyboards, pointing devices and their role in the development of CTS. They also compared several keyboards with respect to design of keyswitch to reduce force and its effect on carpal tunnel pressure. They stated that "ergonomic" keyboards change the musculoskeletal region exposed to risk, instead of eliminating hazardous postures.

Increased hours of computer use, perceived stress levels and workstation factors have also been found to be associated with upper extremity musculoskeletal pain. Evans and Patterson (2000) conducted an epidemiological field study on 170 subjects from Hong Kong workplaces in order to determine the incidence of neck and shoulder pain in a non-secretarial population of computer users. They tested the hypothesis that poor typing skill, hours of computer use, tension score and poor workstation setup are associated with neck and shoulder complaints. Sixty five percent of subjects recorded pain. Through regression analysis, they found that tension score and gender were the only factors to predict neck and shoulder pain.

Westgaard (2000) mentioned about three themes on the work-related musculoskeletal complaints in the coming years. He listed these three themes as risk analysis of low-level biomechanical exposures, risk analysis of low-level psychosocial exposure and implementation of ergonomic intervention.

In their study, Fogleman and Lewis (2002) studied the risk factors associated with the self-reported musculoskeletal discomfort in a population of video display terminal (VDT) operators. They collected data via a survey from 292 VDT users, and asked to report on symptoms for six body regions, as well as job requirement information, demographic information, and non-occupational hobbies. They constructed factor analysis to determine descriptive information and logistic regression to estimate the risk. Their results indicated that there is a statistically significant increased risk of discomfort on each of the body regions (head and eyes, neck and upper back, lower back, shoulders, elbows and forearms, and hands and wrists) as the number of hour of keyboard use increases. Moreover, their results showed that improper monitor and keyboard position were significantly associated with head/eye and shoulder/back discomfort, respectively.

Szeto et al. (2005) compared the EMG changes and discomforts experienced by a symptomatic and an asymptomatic group of workers when they were challenged by the physical stressors of increased typing speed and increased typing force. They divided the respondents into 2 groups, 21 female office worker in the Case Group, and 20 in the Control Group. The respondents were asked to participate a typing test for 20 minutes in 3 conditions; normal, faster, and harder. The Case group showed trends for higher muscle activities in all three conditions in both upper trapezius and cervical erector spinae muscles. There were greater increases in muscle activities in both groups under "faster" condition, implying that increasing the typing speed was a more difficult demand. They further divided the Case Group into High and Low groups. They realized that it was mainly the High group that showed the greatest changes in terms of muscle activities and discomforts.

Shuval and Donchin (2005) examined the relationship between ergonomic risk factors and upper extremity musculoskeletal symptoms in VDT workers, by taking into account individual and work organizational factors, and stress. Their data was derived from a questionnaire responded by 84 workers from computer programmers, managers, administrators, and marketing specialists, while ergonomic data were collected through two direct observations via rapid upper limb assessment (RULA) method. Their results of RULA observations indicated that excessive postural loading with no employee in acceptable postures. Hand/wrist/finger symptoms were related to the RULA arm/wrist score (in a logistic regression model) as well as working with a VDT between 7.1 and 9 hours per day. Neck/shoulder symptoms were related to: gender (female), working more than 10 hours per day, working for more than 2 years in a hi-tech company, and being uncomfortable at the workstation.

Dennerlein and Johnson (2006) studied the differences in biomechanical risk factors across different computer tasks: typing text, completing an html-based form with text fields, editing text within a document, sorting and resizing objects in a graphics task and browsing and navigating a series of intranet web pages through participation of 30 touch-typist adults (15 females, and 15 males). Their results indicated that keyboard-intensive tasks were associated with less neutral wrist postures, larger wrist velocities and accelerations and larger dynamic forearm muscle activity. Mouse-intensive tasks (graphics and web page browsing) were associated with less neutral shoulder postures and less variability in forearm muscle activity, larger range of motion and larger velocities and acceleration of the upper arm. Additionally, their results suggested that comparing different types of computer work demonstrates that mouse use is prevalent in most computer tasks and is associated with more constrained and non-neutral postures of the wrist and shoulder compared to keyboard.

Flodgren et al. (2007) assessed the wrist kinetics (range of motion, mean position, velocity and mean power frequency in radial/ulnar deviation, flexion/extension, and pronation/supination) associated with performing a mouse-operated computerized task involving painting rectangles on a computer screen. Furthermore, they evaluated the effects of the painting task on subjective perception of fatigue and wrist position sense. Their results showed that the painting task required constrained wrist movements, and repetitive movements of about the same magnitude as those performed in mouse-operated design tasks. In addition, their results showed that the painting task induced a perception of muscle fatigue in the upper extremity (Borg CR-scale: 3.5, $p<0.001$) and caused a reduction in the position sense accuracy of the wrist (error before: 4.6°, error after: 5.6°, $p<0.05$). This standardized painting task appears suitable for studying relevant risk factors, and therefore it offers a potential for investigating the pathophysiological mechanisms behind musculoskeletal disorders related to computer mouse use.

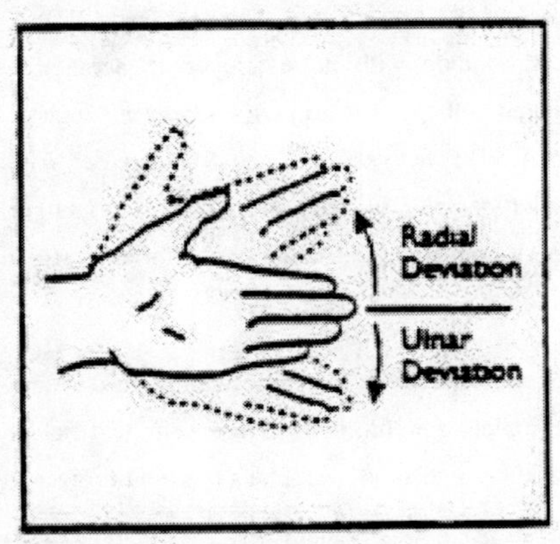

Figure 4. Radial and Ulnar Deviations

Work related musculoskeletal disorders (WMSDs) in the shoulder/neck area are a common and increasing problem among European computer workers, especially women. Thorn et al. (2007) studied the long-term low-level workloads with low degree of muscle rest which results in a potential risk factor for developing WMSDs. Their study on female computer users (age 45–65 years) in Denmark and Sweden investigated if subjects with self-reported neck/shoulder complaints (cases, $N = 35$) show less trapeziusmuscle relative rest time (RRT) than controls ($N = 44$) when performing standardised short-term computer work tasks in controlled laboratory conditions. They recorded surface electromyography (EMG) signals bilaterally from the upper trapezius muscles during a type, edit, precision and colour word stress task. Their results showed that on the average, 15 of the cases and 18 of the controls showed analysable EMG files per task. For the color word stress task, their results showed lower RRT values and higher 10th percentile RMS amplitude levels among cases compared to controls. Furthermore, their results indicated an increased motor response to a psychological stressor among subjects with self-reported neck/shoulder complaints.

Nag et al. (2008) examined the effects of forearm and wrist supports on the upper extremity postures in computer keying tasks and associated EMG activity of arm and back muscles (N=8). In their study, four positions were forearms unsupported (floating) and supported, wrists supported by bead packed (WR1) and gel-filled (WR2) wrist rest. Moreover, the right and left elbow extensions were 65° and 68°, respectively, in unsupported forearms. Their findings indicated bilateral elbow extension increased with the forearm/wrist supports and mostly, the elbow was maintained at around 90° or greater. The wrist extension was decreased with forearm/wrist supports over the unsupported condition. The results also indicated that the forearm support significantly reduced the activity of forearm extensor digitorum, i.e., right ($F_{(1, 47)}$=12.19,p<0.01) and left ($F_{(1, 47)}$=5.38, p<0.05) and upper trapezius muscles over the floating posture. Wrist rests was observed to increase load on the upper trapezius; the activities of flexor digitorum superficialis and erector spinae were observed to be close to the resting EMG activity for both forearm and/or wrist support. Their concern was the type of wrist rests and their study indicated that the gel filled wrist rest was advantageous in reducing the forearm muscle load, in comparison to the bead packed cushions.

Although there has been extensive research about the kinematics of the neck, arm, and wrist during computer keyboarding, there is almost no information concerning the kinematics of the fingers, thumbs, and hands. Baker et al. (2007) established normative values of the kinematics of thefingers and hands during computer keyboard use. They described the angles, angular velocities, and angular accelerations of the metacarpophalangeal joints and proximal interphalangeal joints for the right and left hands of 20 computer keyboard users during a word-processing task. They also defined and examined a new kinematic variable for computer keyboard use, hand/wrist displacement, is also. Hand/wrist displacement refers to the translational movements of the hands in which the entire hand is repositioned to strike the keys. They captured kinematics of both hands of the keyboard users using a three-dimensional motion capture system. Their findings illustrated that metacarpophalangeal joint kinematics in flexion/extension and abduction/adduction were reported during typing. Proximal interphalangeal joint kinematics in flexion/extension were also reported. The means and standard deviations for finger postures, velocities and acceleration were generally not significantly different between the right and left hands, with the exception of the 1st digit (thumb). Hand/wrist displacement was significantly different between the right and left hands for side to side movements.

Two-button computer mouse users may exhibit sustained, static finger lifting behaviors to prevent inadvertent activations by avoiding finger pressure on the buttons, which leads to prolonged, static finger extensor muscle loading. McLoone and Dennerlein (2008) observed one hundred graduate students during normal computer work in a university computer facility to qualify and quantify the prevalence of lifted finger behaviors and extended finger postures, as well as wrist/forearm and grip behavior, during specific mouse activities. Their results indicated that the highest prevalence observed were 48% of the students lifted their middle finger during mouse drag activities, and 23% extended their middle finger while moving the mouse. In addition, during their study 98% of the students rested their wrist and forearm (77%) or wrist only (21%) on the workstation surface, and 97% had an extended wrist posture (15°–30°) when using the mouse. The potential applications of their findings include future computer input device designs to reduce finger lifting behavior and exposures to risk factors of hand / forearm musculoskeletal pain.

David et al. (2008) described the development and evaluation of the Quick Exposure Check (QEC), which is an observational tool developed for Occupational Safety and Health

(OSH) practitioners to assess exposure to risks for work-related musculoskeletal disorders and provide a basis for ergonomic interventions. Their tool was based on epidemiological evidence and investigations of OSH practitioners' aptitudes for undertaking assessments. It has been tested, modified and validated using simulated and workplace tasks, in two phases of development, with participation of 206 practitioners. The QEC allows the four main body areas to be assessed and involves practitioners and workers in the assessment. Through trials, they have determined its usability, intra- and inter-observer reliability, and validity which show it is applicable to a wide range of working activities. Their tool focused primarily on physical workplace factors, but also includes the evaluation of psychosocial factors. Tasks can normally be assessed within 10 min. It has a scoring system, and exposure levels have been proposed to guide priorities for intervention. Their QEC can contribute to a holistic assessment of all the elements of a work system.

Szeto and Sham (2008) investigated the effects of different angled positions of the display screen on neck–shoulder muscle activities. They recruited a group of healthy painfree university students (10 males and 10 females) and they examined muscle activities in the cervical erector spinae (CES) and upper trapezius (UT) muscles. Each of their subjects performed typing tasks for 20 min with a central screen position (CP), angled left position (ALP), and angled right position (ARP). Their results showed median muscle activities were generally higher activities in CES compared to UT. They found significant increases in ipsilateral CES and contralateral UT muscles in both ALP and ARP. They had also significant increases in subjective discomfort scores in ALP (p=0.003) and ARP (p=0.009) compared to CP. Their results showing higher muscle activities with angled screen positions indicated that greater biomechanical exposure that may in turn contribute to musculoskeletal disorders, especially with prolonged computer use.

Several ergonomic studies have estimated computer work duration using registration software. In these studies, an arbitrary pause definition (Pd; the minimal time between two computer events to constitute a pause) is chosen and the resulting duration of computer work is estimated. In order to uncover the relationship between the used pause definition and the computer work duration (PWT), Slijper et al. (2008) used registration software to record usage patterns of 571 computer users across almost 60,000 working days. For a large range of Pds (1–120 s), they found a shallow, log-linear relationship between PWT and Pds. Their results showed that for keyboard and mouse use, a second-order function fitted the data best. We found that these relationships were dependent on the amount of computer work and subject characteristics.

Computer display height and desk design to allow forearm support are two critical design features of workstations for information technology tasks. However there is currently no 3D description of head andneck posture with different computer display heights and no direct comparison to paper based information technology tasks. There is also inconsistent evidence on the effect of forearm support on posture and no evidence on whether these features interact. In their study, Straker et al. (2008) compared the 3D head, neck andupper limb postures of 18 male and 18 female young adults whilst working with different display and desk design conditions. Their results show that there was no substantial interaction between display height and desk design, and lower display heights increased head and neck flexion with more spinal asymmetry when working with paper. Furthermore the curved desk, designed to provide forearm support, increased scapula elevation / protraction and shoulder flexion / abduction.

Since musculoskeletal disorders of the upper extremities are believed to be associated with repetitive excessive muscle force production in the hands, understanding the time-dependent muscle forces during key tapping is essential for exploring the mechanisms of disease initiation and development. In their study, Wu et al. (2008) have simulated the time-dependent dynamic loading in the muscle/tendons in an index fingerduring tapping. They developed index finger model using a commercial software package AnyBody, which contains seven muscle/tendons that connect the three phalangeal finger sections. Their simulations indicate that the ratios of the maximal forces in flexor digitorum superficialis (FS) and flexor digitorum profundus (FP)tendons to the maximal force at the fingertip are 0.95 and 2.9, respectively, which agree well with recently published experimental data. Their results showed that the time sequence of the finger muscle activation predicted in the current study was consistent with the EMG data in the literature.

Ferrigno et al. (2009) examined the effect of wrist orthoses on the electromyography activities of the extensor carpi ulnaris, flexor digitorum superficialis, and fibers of the upper trapezius muscles during computer work. They designed a randomized, 3×2 factorial design: orthoses (no orthosis, wearing a custom-made orthosis, wearing a commercial orthosis) and tasks (typing, using the mouse). The participants in their study were selected among healthy university students (N=23), ranging from 18 to 26 years of age. Study volunteers performed standardized tasks such as typing and using the mouse while wearing 1 of 2 types of wrist orthoses or no orthosis. They used surface electromyography and considered 100% maximum voluntary contraction to represent the amplitude of electromyographic activity. They observed a significant increase in the electromyographic activity of the trapezius ($P<.05$) with the use of orthoses. Their results indicated there was no significant difference in the activities of the flexor digitorum superficialis or extensor carpi ulnaris in participants who typed with or without orthoses ($P>.05$). However, when the participants used the mouse, the extensor muscle presented an increase in activity with both orthoses, and the same pattern was observed in the flexor muscle when the volunteers used the custom-made orthosis. Their findings showed that wrist orthoses affected the muscle activities in the upper limbs of healthy adults who were using a computer. Furthermore, electromyographic activity increased in the trapezius when the subjects used either type of orthosis, and they observed the same pattern in the extensor carpi ulnaris when the subjects used the mouse. The flexor digitorum superficialis presented an increase in activity only when the subjects worked with the mouse and used a custom-made splint.

Won et al. (2009) examined gender differences in upper extremity postures, applied forces, and muscle activity when a computer workstation was adjusted to individual anthropometry according to current guidelines. In their study, fifteen men and fifteen women completed five standardized computer tasks: touch-typing, completing a form, editing text, sorting and resizing graphical objects and navigating intranet pages. Their subjects worked at a height-adjustable workstation with the keyboard on top of the work surface and the mouse to the right. Their subjects repeated the text editing task with the mouse in two other locations: a "high" mouse position, which simulated using a keyboard drawer with the mouse on the primary work surface, and "center" mouse position with the mouse between the keyboard and the body, centered with the body's center line. Surface electromyography measured muscle activity; electrogoniometric and magnetic motion analysis system measured wrist, forearm and upper arm postures; load-cells measured typing forces; and a force-sensing mouse measured applied forces. Their results indicated that relative forces applied to the keyboard, normalized muscle activity of two forearm muscles, range of motion for the wrist and shoulder joints and external rotation of the shoulder were higher for women ($p < 0.05$). When their subjects were dichotomized instead by anthropometry (either large/small shoulder width or arm length), the differences in forces, muscle activity of the shoulder and wrist posture and shoulder posture became more pronounced with smaller subjects having higher values. They indicated that postural differences between the genders increased in the high mouse position and decreased in the center mouse location. Furthermore, their findings showed that when a workstation was adjusted per current guidelines differences in upper extremity force, muscle activity and postural factors still existed between genders.

Samani et al. (2009) evaluated effects of active and passive pauses and investigate the distribution of the trapezius surface electromyographic (SEMG) activity during computer mouse work. Twelve healthy male subjects performed four sessions of computer work for 10 min in one day, with passive (relax) and active (30% maximum voluntary contraction of shoulder elevation) pauses given every 2 min at two different work paces (low/high). Bipolar SEMG from four parts of the trapezius muscle was recorded. The relative rest time was higher for the lower parts compared with the upper of the trapezius ($p < 0.01$). The centroid of exposure variation analysis (EVA) along the time axis was lower during the computer work with active pause compared with passive one ($p < 0.05$). The results of this study revealed (i) lower rest time for the upper parts of trapezius compared with the lower parts, in line with previous clinical findings, (ii) active pauses contributed to a more variable muscle activity pattern during computer work that might have functional implications with respect to work-related musculoskeletal disorders.

Østensvik et al. (2009) evaluated different aspects of muscle activity patterns associated with musculoskeletal discomfort/pain. They conducted surface electromyography (sEMG) of the right upper trapezius and the right extensor digitorum muscles continuously during one working day in 19 male forest machine operators driving harvesters, 20 driving forwarders and 20 researchers at the Forest Research Institute. They rated perceived discomfort/pain in the right side of the neck and the right forearm in morning, noon and afternoon with Borg's CR-10 scale. They analyzed static, median and peak levels of muscle activity and the number and they calculated total duration of EMG gaps (muscular rest). Sustained low-level muscle activity (SULMA) was defined as continuous muscle activity above 0.5% of the maximal EMG activity quantified into 10 periods of predetermined duration intervals from 1.6 to 5 s up to above 20 min. They presented the number of SULMA periods within each interval and as cumulative periods above the already determined levels. Their operators handled control levers seated in a fixed position while the researchers performed mainly PC work and other varied tasks. Their results showed that a positive correlation was found between discomfort/pain in the right upper trapezius muscle region in the afternoon and cumulative SULMA periods above 10 min duration, and a negative correlation to cumulative SULMA periods also including the short durations. There were no specified patterns for discomfort/pain in the right extensor digitorum or for the other EMG measurements. All EMG measurements distinguished to some extent between the occupational groups, especially between machine operators driving harvesters and researchers. Furthermore, they found that number of SULMA periods longer than 10 min per hour was positively correlated, and predominantly short periods were negatively correlated, to complaints in the neck region. They stated that this seems promising in order to find duration limits for sustained low-level muscle activity as a risk factor for musculoskeletal disorders.

Jacobs et al. (2009) suggested that university students self-reporting experiencing musculoskeletal discomfort with computer use were similar to levels reported by adult workers. Their objective was to determine how university students use notebook computers and to determine what ergonomic strategies might be effective in reducing self-reported musculoskeletal discomfort in this population. They randomly assigned two hundred and eighty-nine university students to one of three towers by the university's Office of Housing participated in this study. The results of their investigation showed a significant reduction in self-reported notebook computer-related discomfort from pre- and post-survey in participants who received notebook computer accessories and in those who received accessories and participatory ergonomics training. They indicated that there was a significant increase in post-survey rest breaks. Furthermore, there was a significant correlation between self-reported computer usage and the amount measured using computer usage software (odometer).

Straker et al. (2009) indicated that the use of computers by children has increased rapidly, however few studies have addressed factors which may reduce musculoskeletal stress during computer use by children. This study quantified the postural and muscle activity effects of providing forearm support when children used computers. Twelve male and 12 female children (10–12 years) who regularly used computers were recruited. Activities were completed using a computer with two workstation configurations, one of which provided for forearm support on the desk surface. 3D posture was analysed using an infra-red motion analysis system. Surface EMG was collected from five muscle groups in the neck/shoulder region and right upper limb. Providing a support surface resulted in more elevated and flexed upper limbs. The use of forearm or wrist support was associated with reduced muscle activity for most muscle groups. Muscle activity reductions with support were of sufficient magnitude to be clinically meaningful. The provision of a supporting surface for the arm is therefore likely to be useful for reducing musculoskeletal stresses associated with computing tasks for children.

Past research on work-related musculoskeletal disorders (WMSD) has frequently examined the activity of neck–shoulder muscles such as upper trapezius (UT) and cervical erector spinae (CES) during typing tasks. Increased electromyographic activity in these postural stabilising muscles has been consistently found in chronic neck pain patients under different physically stressful conditions. Szeto et al. (2009) compared muscle activity when female office workers with chronic neck pain ($n = 39$) and asymptomatic controls ($n = 34$) adopted two resting postures: (1) with hands on laps versus; and (2) hands on a keyboard. Their results indicated that resting hands on keyboard elicited significantly increased muscle activity in the right upper trapezius (UT) of subjects with high discomforts ($n = 22$), similar to that observed during actual typing. In contrast, the asymptomatic controls showed no difference in muscle activity between the resting postures. Their results suggested that altered muscle activation patterns were triggered by some anticipatory task demand associated with a task-specific position in some individuals.

Korhan and Mackieh (2010) investigated the effect of musculoskeletal discomfort and their frequencies associated with the use of computers has not received. Their work presented the findings of a risk assessment model through a scientific research to determine the effect of discomfort factors that contribute to musculoskeletal disorders resulting from intensive use of computers in the workplaces. They gave a questionnaire to 130 intensive computer users working for the university sector in Cyprus. They developed a list of significant predictor variables for musculoskeletal disorders to assess and analyze workplace ergonomics, worker attitudes and experiences on computer keyboard and mouse. The main focus of their research was to seek and provide evidence that symptoms of musculoskeletal discomfort and the frequency of these symptoms are significant in the development of Work Related Musculoskeletal Disorders (WRMSDs). Their study provides the evidence that, ache and pain are the most common types of discomforts in all body regions. They showed that the discomforts were more pronounced at neck, shoulder, upper back, hand/wrist, and lower back regions. They also validated the risk factors determined by their risk assessment model through ANOVA of the sEMG records for the control and test groups. Their findings indicated that for each test group respondent, the mean musculoskeletal strain experienced differs in time, but the same is not true for the control group.

8. Postures

In order to improve the work performance; workplace, working posture, and discomfort are needed to be justified. Liao and Drury (2000) demonstrated the interactions between workplace, work duration, discomfort, working posture, as well as performance in a 2 hour typing task. They used three levels of keyboard heights to investigate the effects on working posture, and discomfort (perceived body part discomfort) and performance (typing speed, error rate and error correction rate). Their results showed that the interrelationships among posture-comfort-performance were supported. Moreover, keyboard height had effects o working posture adopted.

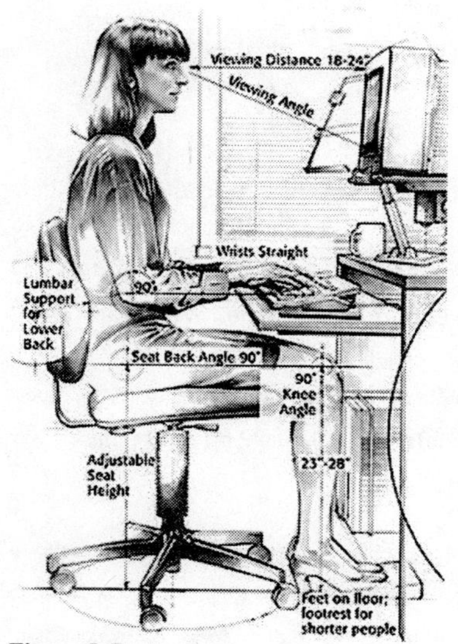

Figure 5. Posture

Babski-Reeves et al. (2005) studied the effects of monitor height and chair type on low back and neck muscle activity, perceived level of discomfort, and posture shifts. They investigated if chairs at opposing ends of their price spectrum differ in physiological benefits. Their findings indicated that the interaction of monitor height and chair type significantly affects the loads placed on the human body. Task demands were also played an important role in the loads placed on the body, posture fixity, and level of discomfort reported. Therefore, they stated that the location of VDT equipment and chair selection should be based on task demands to minimize static loading and discomfort.

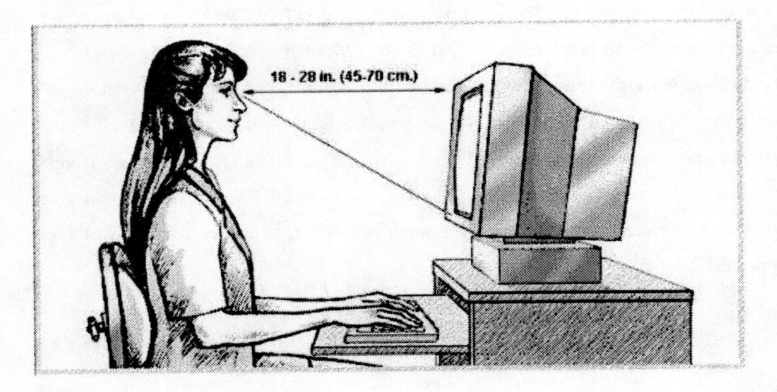

Figure 6. Monitor height

Laptop computers were introduced into the workplace for reasons of portability. However laptop computer screens and keyboards are joined, and therefore they are unable to be adjusted separately in terms of screen height and distance, and keyboard height and distance. Straker et al. (1997) studied the postural implications of using a laptop computer. Their results showed that there were significantly greater neck flexion and head tilt with laptop use. Trunk, shoulder, elbow, wrist, and scapula did not show any statistical differences. Additionally, the average discomfort experienced after using the laptop for 20 minutes was not significantly greater.

Straker and Mekhora (1999) investigated the effects of monitor placement in a group of normal subjects. Ten male and ten female subjects within the working age range volunteered to perform a computing task for 20 min in two different VDU monitor placement conditions; high monitor position (HMP) and a low monitor position (LMP). Postural angles (gaze, head, neck, and trunk), normalized electromyography (upper trapezius and cervical and thoracic erector spinae), discomfort (upper body), and individual preference for monitor placement were determined. Their results indicated that the gaze, head, neck, and trunk angles in the LMP were significantly greater (more flexed) than those in the HMP. There was a trend for lower levels of electromyographic (EMG) activity for trapezius in the HMP. There were significantly lower levels of EMG activity for cervical and thoracic erector spinae in HMP. The results of their study suggested that subjects may use a less flexed head, neck and trunk posture and less cervical and erector spinae muscle activity when working with a HMP.

Notebook computers users reported more constrained posture and higher neck muscle activities that those of desktop computers. Jonai et al. (2002) investigated the effects of liquid crystal display (LCD) tilt angle of a notebook computer on posture, muscle activities and somatic complaints in 10 subjects. They found that at the tilt angle of 100^0, the subjects were noted to have relatively less neck flexion. Also, the static neck extensor muscle activity was observed to be the lowest at this tilt angle. Their results strongly suggested that the ergonomic features and problems attributable to notebook computers are distinct from the desktop computers.

There has been substantial research carried out to evaluate the effects of working on a VDT, keyboard and input device using desktop PCs. In response to discomfort, poor posture and restricted movement due to the inability to separate the keyboard and VDT in laptop PCs, "laptopstations" have been introduced to the market. Berkhout et al. (2003) studied the effect of using laptopstation and a laptop PC and how this difference in work setup affected the mechanical load on the neck, and productivity. Their results indicated that there was a significant ($p<0.005$) difference with the use of the laptopstation resulting in decreased torque, less perceived strain at the neck and a higher productivity score. Additionally, their results confirm the importance of adjustable work tools that recognize anthropometric differences and biomechanics to meet the needs of individual customers during continuous VDT work.

Muss and Hedge (1999), worked on the effects of an alternative keyboard design, a vertical split-keyboard with attached, width-adjustable palm supports on dynamic wrist posture, self-reports of fatigue and discomfort, and typing performance. The results are then compared to a traditional keyboard, and it was observed that the vertical split-keyboard design reduced ulnar deviation and wrist extension as compared to the traditional keyboard, but did not improve user comfort and typing performance as compared to a traditional keyboard.

Marshall et al. (1999) constructed a quantitative analysis of the effects of complex wrist/forearm posture on range of motion. For each of the sample groups, 35 men and 19 women, they measured 24 different wrist deviations (6 flexion, 6 extension, 6 radial deviation, 6 ulnar deviation). Their study revealed that combinations of wrist/forearm postures have significant effects on wrist range of motion, where the largest effects were observed from those of wrist flexion/exertion on radial deviation range of motion.

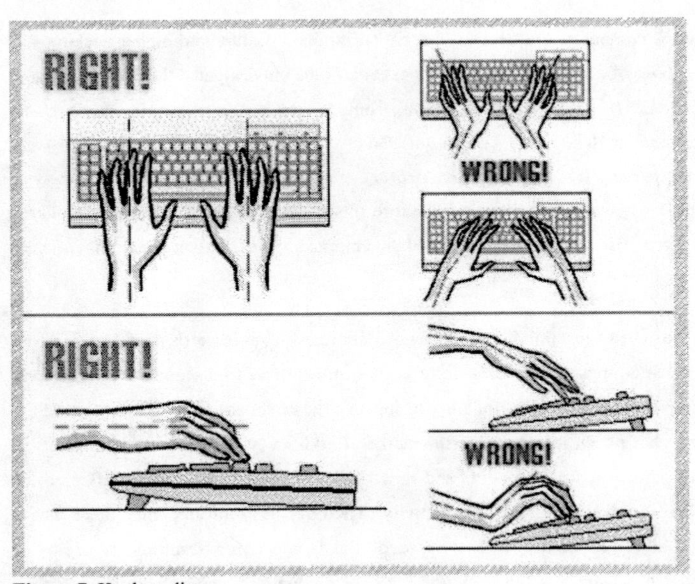

Figure 7. Keyboarding

Simoneau et al. (1999) performed a comprehensive investigation to document wrist and forearm postures of users of conventional computer keyboards. They tested 90 healthy, experienced clerical workers with electromechanical goiometers to measure wrist and forearm position and range of motion for both upper extremities while typing. Their results indicated that for alphabetic typing task, the left wrist showed significantly greater ($p<0.01$) mean ulnar deviation ($15.0^0 \pm 7.7^0$) and extension ($21.2^0 \pm 8.8^0$) than the right wrist ($10.1^0 \pm 7.2^0$ and $17.0^0 \pm 7.4^0$ for ulnar deviation and extension respectively). On the other hand, the right forearm had greater mean pronation ($65.6^0 \pm 8.3^0$) than the left forearm ($62.2^0 \pm 10.6^0$). They found out that there were minimal functional differences in the postures of the wrists and forearms between alphabetic and alphanumeric typing tasks.

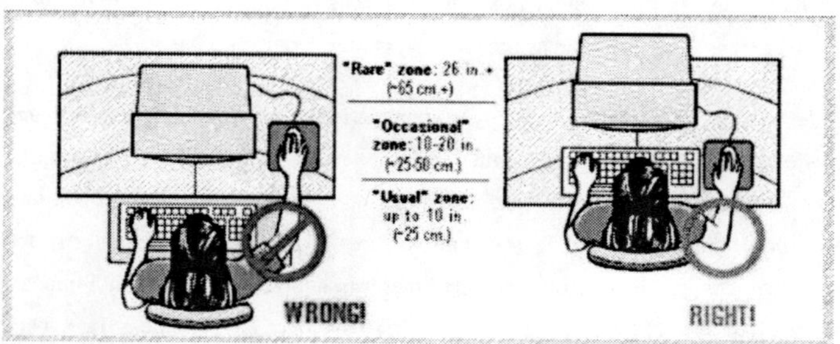

Figure 8. Forearm position

Marklin et al. (1999) conducted a study on 90 experienced office workers to determine how commercially available alternative computer keyboards affected wrist and forearm posture. They tested split flixed angle, split adjustable angle, and vertically inclined (tilted or tended). Their results showed that when set up correctly, commercially available split keyboards reduced mean ulnar deviation of the right and left wrists from 12^0 to within 5^0 of a neutral position compared with a conventional keyboard. Additionally, split keyboards place the wrist closer to a neutral posture in the radial/ulnar plane reduces the ulnar deviation of the wrist, which is an occupational risk factor of WRMSDs.

Simoneau and Marklin (2001) conducted a research to determine the systematic effect varying the slope angle of a computer keyboard along with varying keyboard height have on wrist extension while typing. The participants typed on a keyboard whose slope was adjusted to $+15^0$, $+7.5^0$, 0^0, -7.5^0, and -15^0. The results showed that as keyboard slope angle moved downward from $+15^0$ to -15^0, mean wrist extension decreased approximately 13^0, which means wrist extension angles of $+15^0$ or less are beneficial compared with wrist extension greater than $+15^0$ and would reduce the risk of WRMSDs.

Another research on high static loading of the forearm extensor musculature during keying tasks was conducted by Keir and Wells (2002). They simulate the human finger to determine the force contributions during a static index finger press at several wrist postures. The results indicated that greater than 25% of maximal exertion is required of the wrist extensors when the wrist is extended to 30^0, and states that the increased moment contribution from passive forces of the extrinsic finger flexor muscles was responsible for the majority of the increased wrist extensor contribution as the wrist was extended.

Fernandez et al. (1999) investigated the implementation of an arm support system and its effect on the level of the pain and/or discomfort experienced by subjects during a computer typing task. The 15 male student subjects performed the required task under four conditions; no arm support, arm support attached to the chair, ergorest articulation arm supports, and counter-balanced arm slings. Their results indicated that arm supports significantly impacted comfort, effort required, rate of perceived exertion (RPE), EMG activity, and heart rate. They concluded that in computer work tasks, an arm support system would be recommended to minimize effort and RPE, and to maximize comfort.

Park et al. (2000) proposed a new concept VDT workstation chair with an adjustable keyboard and mouse support to minimize the physical discomfort and the risk of CDTs at work sites. Based upon the result of 3-D graphical simulations, a mock-up chair was constructed with an adjustable keyboard/mouse support directly attached to the chair body. They constructed an experiment to compare the new workstation chair to a conventional computer chair without a keyboard and mouse support by measuring muscle fatigue and subjective discomfort. Their statistical results indicated that the new concept VDT chair generally improved subjective comfort level and reduced fatigue in the finger flexor/extensor and the low back muscles.

Vergara and Page (2001) conducted a study to analyze the causes of lumbar discomfort while sitting on a chair, by analyzing the relationship of lumbar curvature, pelvic inclination and their mobilities with discomfort. They performed an experiment with healthy subjects, in which comfort, postural and mobility parameters have been measured. Their relationship has been analyzed with multivariate analysis. Factorial analysis has been used to represent all the correlated variables measured. Logistic regression and discriminant analyses have been used to classify discomfort/absence of discomfort. The results show that great changes of posture are a good indicator of discomfort, and that lordotic postures with forward leaned pelvis and low mobility are the principal causes of the increase of discomfort.

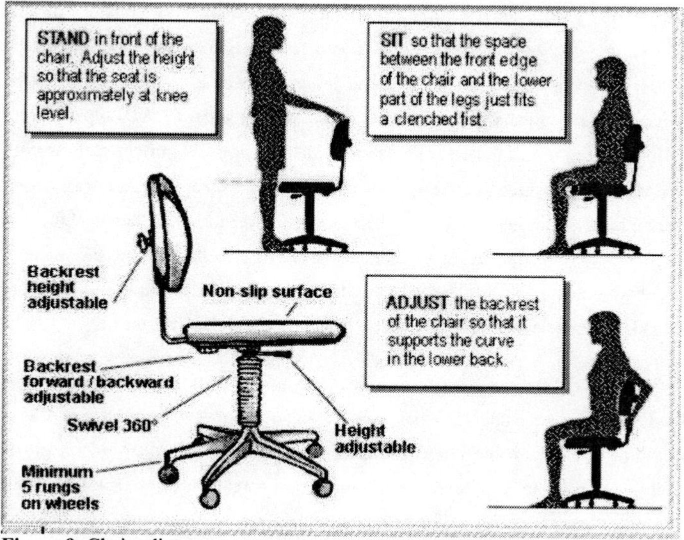

Figure 9. Chair adjustment

Carey and Gallwey (2001) investigated the effects of exertion, pace and level of simple and combined flexion/extension and radial/ulnar deviation of the wrist on discomfort for simple repetitive exertions. Eight male subjects participated in the study and the level of exertion and angular deviation were defined relative to the maximum strength and range of motion of the subjects, respectively. They found out that extreme flexion caused higher discomfort than the other simple types of deviation, and the combination of flexion and ulnar deviation resulted in higher discomfort than the other types of combined deviation. Moreover, exertion was the most significant factor, followed by level of deviation and then pace.

Gerard et al. (2002) worked on a laboratory study to determine the effects of work pace on typing force, electromyographic activity and subjective discomfort. The findings include as the participants typed faster, their typing force and finger flexor and extensor electromyographic activity increased linearly. Their findings showed that the relative pace of typing is more important than actual typing speed with regard to discomfort and muscle activity.

Tepper et al. (2003) investigated whether an ergonomic computer device, characterized by an inclined working area and keyboard localization close to the screen (the Up-Line), decreases the muscle activity of the upper trapezius muscle. In a crossover design 19 healthy subjects and 19 patients with Whiplash Associated Disorder (WAD) typed during 10 min at the Up-Line and at a standard workstation with 15 min of rest in between. During typing surface EMG was measured of the trapezius muscle. They asked subjects to rate sitting comfort and complaints. Although most subjects subjectively preferred the Up-Line, on average, they found out no significant differences in muscle activity between the two workstations for both patients and healthy subjects. Individually in 5 healthy subjects (25%) and in 6 patients (31%) muscle activity was lower when working at the Up-Line.

Cook and Burgess-Limerick (2004) examined the effect of three different postures during keyboard use: forearm support, wrist support and floating (no support, used as a reference condition), in order to understand the effect of forearm support on wrist posture. Electromyography was used to monitor neck, shoulder and forearm muscle activity. Their findings indicate that typing with upper extremity support in conjunction with a wrist may be preferable to the floating posture.

Cook et al. (2004) examined the effect of wrist rest use on wrist posture during forearm support. They conducted an experiment on 15 subjects to examine muscle activity and wrist postures during keyboard and mouse tasks in two conditions (wrist rest, no wrist rest). Their results showed that there were no significant differences for right wrist flexion/extension between use of a wrist rest and no wrist rest for keyboard or mouse use. Moreover, left writ extension was significantly higher without a wrist rest than with a wrist rest during keyboard use. Additionally, they found out that there were no differences with respect to use of a wrist rest for the left or right hand for ulnar deviation for keyboard or mouse use.

Supporting the forearm on the work surface during keyboard operation may increase comfort, decrease muscular load of the neck and shoulders, and decrease the time spent in ulnar deviation. Cook and Burgess-Limerick (2004) investigated the musculoskeletal discomfort effects of using forearm support in intensive computer users in a call center. A controlled study was conducted on 59 subjects; group 1 with forearm support, group 2 with "floating" posture. Their results showed that there were significantly fewer reports of discomfort in the neck and back, although the difference between the groups was not statistically significant. Therefore, their findings indicate that forearm support may be preferable to the "floating" posture for computer workstation setup.

Musculoskeletal problems reported by school children using computers have often been linked to bad posture. In their study, Robbins et al. (2009) investigated whether posture education affects the reported prevalence of musculoskeletal symptoms amongst secondary school children using computers. They designed a prospective blinded randomized controlled trial. The participants in their study were seventy-one school children aged 11–12 years divided into intervention ($n = 37$) and control ($n = 34$) groups. They assessed both groups received posture training delivered by teachers at the school and on their knowledge of correct posture. Then they gave a follow-up lesson 1 week later during which the intervention group also received automated posture warnings and tips on their personal computers. They noted the prevalence and severity of musculoskeletal symptoms were measured at the start of the study and at the start and end of the follow-up lesson and any differences between the two groups found over the course of the 60 min follow-up lesson. Their results indicated that by the end of the follow-up lesson, the mean visual analogue pain scale representation of the degree of discomfort due to the musculoskeletal problems fell significantly from 1.53 to 0.39 for the intervention group, while that for the control group only fell from 1.23 to 1.13 (non-significant). Furthermore, their overall incidence of musculoskeletal problems in the intervention group showed a greater trend towards reduction, falling significantly from 32.4% to 5.4% compared with the control group, which fell from 29.4% to 20.59% (non-significant).

9. Psychosocial Factors

Work-related musculoskeletal disorders (MSD) have a multifactorial etiology that includes not only physical stressors but also psychosocial risk factors, such as job strain, social support at work, and job dissatisfaction. Once an injury has occurred, psychosocial factors, such as depression and maladaptive pain responses, are pivotal in the transition from acute to chronic pain and the development of disability (Menzel, Nancy N., 2007).

Hudiburg, Pashaj, and Wolfe (1995) reported that preliminary studies have focused more on the outcomes of human-computer interactions and less on the personal characteristics of the computer users. Costa and McCrae (1985) extended the dimensions of personality traits of Eysenck and Eysenck to five broad traits: Neuroticism, Extraversion, Openness to Experience, Agreeableness and Conscientiousness. In order to evaluate the computer use and knowledge of the participants, a research questionnaire was constructed with three scales: the Computer Hassles Scale, SCL-90, and the Big Five Inventory. The Computer Hassles Scale was significantly correlated with somatization or anxiety rating. The Big Five personality traits yielded only a few significant correlations with computer users' stress and stress outcomes. Only Openness was significantly correlated with the Computer Hassles Score. Only Neuroticism was significantly correlated with the somatization or anxiety ratings.

Later in 1996, Hudiburg and Necessary indicated that computer users experience varying degrees of computer stress. Computer use, computer knowledge, self-esteem, level of computer-stress, somatization or anxiety, stressful computer problem were investigated in a research questionnaire to develop coping strategies. The participants were classified as either experiencing high or low levels of computer-stress, according to the data derived from the Computer Hassles Scale. The study suggests that high computer-stress users had lower self-rated computer abilities, lower self-esteem, and higher levels of somatization and anxiety. In contrast, to low computer-stress users, high computer-stress users significantly experienced higher levels confrontive, self-controlling, and accepting responsibility coping strategies in dealing with computer problems.

A continued interest in computer related stress directed Hudiburg to develop the Computer Technology Hassles Scale. A "computer hassle" is a stimulus perceived as a stressor. A survey of 37-item Computer Hassles Scale was constructed to measure the rate the severity of each hassle. The study suggests that the severity of hassles scores on the Computer Hassles Scale were consistently significantly correlated with somatic or anxiety complaints. In regard to this, high and low computer-stress groups were identified according to the severity of hassles scores for the full scale and subscales. The upper quartile was observed to have high computer users' stress. In contrast, the lower quartile was the group having low computer users' stress.

MIT has a continued interest on human-machine interaction. During interaction with computers, humans encounter with unpleasant side effects, which lead to strong, negative emotional states. Frustration, confusion, anger, anxiety can affect not only the interaction itself, but also productivity, learning, social relationships, and overall well-being. A design was conducted by Jonathan Klein at MIT (1999), to study frustration in human subjects by using social, emotional content feedback strategies to help to relieve their emotional state. The results show that social, emotional content interaction with a computer, users experiencing frustration can help to relieve this negative state.

Bongers, Cornelius, Michiel, and Vincent (1993) studied the correlation between psychosocial work factors and musculoskeletal diseases using a qualitative review of medical literature. The data of the study suggests that monotonous work, high-perceived workload, and the press are related to musculoskeletal symptoms. Perceived stress is found to be an intermediary in the growth of musculoskeletal disease. In addition, the study concluded that stress symptoms are often associated with musculoskeletal disease, and more studies indicate that stress symptoms contribute to the development of this disease.

Bo Melin (1997) indicated that psychological stress is not only induced by demands that exceed the individual's mental resources, but also by demands that are too low. The study states that many simple and repetitive work situations lead to common health problems, like musculoskeletal disorders in neck, shoulder and back pain problems. In addition, low job satisfaction elevated psychophysiological stress reactions and lack of relaxation/break seem more important for musculoskeletal problems in some simple and repetitive jobs than poor postures and lifting heavy loads. The data suggests that mental stress induces muscular tension, and that individuals at risk for musculoskeletal disorders are characterized by lack of relaxation/break and elevated physiological arousal in non-work situations.

Preliminary studies have investigated possible risk factors responsible for the development of musculoskeletal disorders (MSDs). This lead Gary W. Allread to investigate the relationship between personality and risk factors for musculoskeletal disorders by focusing on two primary groups of factors, which evolved physical work place demands and psychosocial stressors. These stressors have an influence in producing injury risk and the impact of these risk factors is related with one's personality. Personality research has been conducted to understand whether individuals better matched with their physical work environment exhibited less psychosocial strain and lower MSDs risk than those more mismatched with their workplace. The results indicated that individuals' responses to many psychosocial indices were related to their personalities. It is concluded that employees whose personalities were more mismatched with their work environment exhibited higher psychosocial strain. Moreover. Trunk muscle activities and predicted spinal loading were found to be influenced by both psychosocial stress and the subject's personality.

Hyunsuk Suh (2000) indicated that, with the introduction of computer-based technology to the office work environment, the concern for adverse mental and physical health outcomes of office workers became a primary issue in job stress research. Complaints of visual discomfort, muscular aches, and psychological disturbances arouse by unhealthy working conditions with the increased dependency on technology. Preliminary researches have studied the linkage between work factors to musculoskeletal discomfort and stress. It was suggested that these factors are combined in a system to create stress-inducing situations, which result in musculoskeletal disorders. A research was constructed to test the conceptual model of risk perception in the work organization. The model assumes that individual's perception of work-related risk has a significant impact on the outcome of stress. A tool for measuring risk perception, with its degree of contribution to musculoskeletal discomfort and stress explored the primary tasks in the study.

In their study. Pascale, Smith, and Haims (1999) proposed several pathways for a theoretical relationship between job stress and work-related musculoskeletal disorders (WRMDs) to support the links among work organization, job stress and WRMDs. These pathways highlight the physiological, psychological, and behavioral reactions to stress that can affect WRMDs directly. A constructed model illustrates that psychosocial work factors (work pressure, lack of control), which can cause stress, might also influence or be related to ergonomic factors such as force, repetition, and posture that have been identified as risk factors for WRMDs. The applications of the research include practitioners taking into account psychosocial work factors and job stress in their efforts to reduce and control WRMDs.

Aaras et al. (1999) studied the musculoskeletal, visual and psychosocial stress in VDU operators before and after multidisciplinary ergonomic intervention. They divided the participants into three groups; two intervention groups (T and S) and one control group (C) of VDU operators. They carried out three serial interventions in the T and S groups, first a lightening system, then new workplaces and last an optometric examination. Their results indicated that the two intervention groups reported significantly improvement of the lightening condition, as well as of the visual conditions and significantly reduced visual discomfort and glare. Additionally, significant reduction of headache was found in one of the intervention groups. Optometric corrections reduced the visual discomfort in both the intervention groups. The control group reported no improvements for any of the health outcomes. Moreover, before the intervention there were no significant differences among the three groups regarding shoulder pain and static trapezius EMG load. Two years after the intervention, a significant reduction of shoulder pain and static trapezius load were reported in the T and S groups, while no such reduction was found in the C group.

Pentti Seppaelae (2001) developed a questionnaire on the use of information technology and stress at work to administer in 3 organizational units of a large municipality. Psychosocial and organizational factors were related to the experiences of psychological stress as well as to musculoskeletal disorders and problems with vision. The occupational groups differed according to the main sources of stress. In regression analyses, workload and haste, management and work atmosphere, work demands, defects of the workplace, and gender explained 42% of the experience of mental stress and anxiety. Workload and haste, management and atmosphere, defects of the workplace, hours of daily computer use, and gender explained 25% of the complaints of discomfort of the upper limbs. 19% of the problems with vision were explained by age, workload and haste, defects of the workplace, hours of daily computer use, skills in computer use, and stress related to computer use.

Carayon et al. (2000) proposed several pathways for a theoretical relationship between job stress and WRMSDs. These pathways highlight the physiological, psychological, and behavioral reactions to stress that can affect WRMSDs directly and indirectly. Their model stipulates that psychosocial work factors (e.g. work pressure, lack of control), which can cause stress, might also influence or be related to ergonomic factors such as force, repetition, and posture that have been identified as risk factor for WRMSDs.

Rubenowitz (2000) proposed that the prevalence of musculoskeletal symptoms cannot easily be eliminated by technical measures. However, psychosocial work environment factors should be paid attention. Therefore, he developed and empirically tested interventions aimed at eliminating ergonomic problems based upon six systematic steps are recommended with surveys. He emphasized that attention should be paid not only to physical conditions but also to psychosocial conditions. He later described the most common obstacles to obtaining positive intervention results. He reviewed finally, these were lack of commitment from the manager's point of view, neglecting to engage technicians and employees concerned, ignoring to take psychosocial conditions into consideration, and ignoring the impacts of the proposed changes on the wage system and the organizational system.

Peper et al. (2003) reviewed the ergonomic and psychosocial factors that affect musculoskeletal disorders at the workstation. Thus, they constructed three different methods, where the participants were asked to work on a computer. First was a model of a physiological assessment protocol that incorporated surface-electromyography (SEMG) monitoring while working on a computer. The participants had ergonomic chairs, document holders and foot supports, and obtained an ergonomically comfortable position. They used a typing test, where a word appears directly above an edit box, and the participants were asked to type that given word. SEMG was monitored from four muscle locations. The results showed that there was a significant difference in right forearm extensor-flexor muscle tension and in right upper trapezius muscle tension between type tasks and rest. Also, there was a significant increase in respiration rate from resting to type tasks. Second was a study that showed that participants lack of awareness of their muscle tension as compared to the actual SEMG levels. This time, the keyboard was placed on a tray that could be moved forward or backward and locked into position. The moveable keyboard tray was marked with five positions at 4.5 cm intervals. The participants were monitored during sequential non-typing and typing tasks. Participants rated shoulder, forearm, trapezius and deltoid muscle tensions significantly higher during typing than during non-typing. Their final study illustrated how an intervention program can reduce repetitive strain injury symptoms, decrease respiration rate, and lower SEMG activity. This time, the participants performed the following sequence in two phases, without training and with training: sitting quietly with hands in lap, hand resting on mouse, tracking task (using the mouse), a correcting task (using again the mouse), hand resting on the mouse, and hands resting on lap. The intervention study demonstrated that, the participants could learn to lower trapezius SEMG activity and respiration rate and reduce symptoms of repetitive strain injury.

Sprigg et. al (2007) discussed the demands of the modern office are thought to contribute to the development of musculoskeletal disorders. According to them, for upper body and lower back disorders, these effects were hypothesized to be mediated by psychological strain. They made a study of 936 employees from 22 call centers supports this hypothesis. Using logistic regression and structural equation modeling, they found that the relationship of workload to upper body and lower back musculoskeletal disorders was largely accounted for by job-related strain. This mediating effect was less evident for arm disorders. On the other hand, they showed that job autonomy had neither a direct nor a moderating effect on any musculoskeletal disorder.

In their cross-sectional study of 267 hospital workers from different professions, Wadman and Kjellberg (2007) tested the hypothesis that affective stress responses mediate the effects of the psychosocial work environment on musculoskeletal complaints (MSCs). They analyzed self-reported psychosocial conditions, ergonomic workloads, affective stress and energy responses, and MSCs with a series of logistic regression analyses. Their results showed that psychosocial variables were strongly related to stress and energy, and stress was related to MSCs. Neck and shoulder complaints were more common in the group with high demands and low skill discretion. In their study, this was the only significant relation between psychosocial variables and MSCs that was not explained by their confounding with ergonomic workload. However, they stated that controlling for stress did not substantially reduce or reduce this interaction effect, which would have been the case if it had been mediated (completely or partially) by stress.

10. Physical Factors

Coury et al. (2002) investigated the influence of gender on work-related musculoskeletal disorders in repetitive task. They compared WRMSDs symptoms for female and male workers doing the same repetitive industrial tasks. Logistic regression analysis indicated that symptoms were primarily influenced by the work done. Symptoms were secondarily influenced by gender, job tenure, and age. When compared within the same age group or in the same job tenure, they found that, there was no significant difference in symptoms between male and female workers. Thus, according to them, when confronting poor working conditions, replacements of female workers by male workers is a worthless strategy to control WRMSDs.

Karlqvist et al. (2002) studied the prevalence of musculoskeletal symptoms among male and female VDU operators, and the associations between work-related physical and psychosocial exposures and neck and upper limb symptoms by gender. They collected data on physical and psychosocial exposures and musculoskeletal symptoms by questionnaires. Their results showed that 19% of women (n=785) and 12% of men (n=498) did more than 3 hours of continued computer work without breaks of more than 10 minutes at least twice a week. Men experienced high job strain twice as women. Additionally, a higher proportion of women than men reported symptoms more at least 3 days the preceding month from the upper body. Their results also indicated that duration of computer work was associated with symptoms among both men and women. Only among men, duration of work with a non-keyboard computer input device was associated with symptoms. Only among women, job strain was associated with the symptoms. Time pressure was found to be associated with higher prevalence of symptoms among women. Women experienced higher prevalence of symptoms than men in all body regions and they were more often exposed to physical and psychosocial conditions.

Chaparro et al. (1999) examined the effects of aging on performance and preferences for two computer pointing devices (mouse and trackball). In their study, participants made simple point-and-click and click-and-drag movements to targets of varying distance (96 and 192 mm) and widths (3, 6 and 12 mm). Their results showed that older adults (mean=70) moved more slowly than younger adults (mean=32). Moreover, no age differences were found in movement time or variable error between the two devices. EMG recordings form the forearm flexor and extensor muscles showed no age related differences in between mouse and trackball. However, ratings of perceived exertion (RPE) indicated that older adults perceived greater levels of exertion than younger adults when using the mouse during click-and-drag tasks.

Ferreira and Saldiva (2002) assessed 62 workers engaged in computer-telephone interactive tasks in an active telemarketing center and a telephone call center of an international bank subsidiary in Brazil, by means of a work analysis and a self-administered questionnaire aiming to determine the statistical relationship of ergonomic, organizational and psychosocial characteristics of their jobs with the report of symptoms in neck-shoulder and hand-wrist for more than 7 consecutive days and any time away from work during the current job due to musculoskeletal disorders. They constructed chi-square univariate tests and multiple logistic regression models and found out that active telemarketing operations, duration in the job and the low level of satisfaction with the physical arrangement of the workstation emerged as the factors most related to neck-shoulder and hand-wrist MSD and MSD-induced time away from work. Their study emphasizes the role of psychosocial factors and duration in the job in MSD occurrence and induced absenteeism among workers engaged in computer-telephone interactive tasks.

Balcı and Aghazadeh (2003) introduced the consideration of proper work-rest schedule to help to reduce the musculoskeletal disorders for VDT operators. They studied the comparison work-rest schedules (60 min work/10 min rest, 30 min work/5 min rest, 15 min work/micro-breaks) for VDT operators considering data entry and mental arithmetic tasks. Ten participants were chosen among male college students and the methodology of the study included a discomfort questionnaire and performance measures. Their results indicated that the 15/micro-breaks schedule resulted in significantly lower discomfort in the neck, lower back, and chest than the other schedules. The 30/5 schedule followed by 15/micro-break schedule were found to have the lowest eyestrain and blurred vision. In addition, discomfort in the elbow and arm was found to be lowest with the 15/micro-breaks schedule for the mental arithmetic task. The 15/micro-break schedule resulted in the highest speed, accuracy, and performance for both of the tasks. Moreover, their results showed that the data entry task resulted in significantly increased speed, accuracy, and performance, and lower shoulder and chest discomfort than the mental arithmetic task.

Micro-breaks are scheduled rest breaks taken to prevent the onset or progression of cumulative trauma disorders in the computerized workstation environment. McLean et al. (2001) examined the benefit of micro-breaks by investigating electromyographic signal behavior, perceived discomfort, and worker productivity while individuals performed their usual keying work. Participants provided data from working sessions where they took no breaks, and from working sessions where they took breaks according to their group assignment: micro-breaks at their own discretion (control), micro-breaks at 20 min intervals, and micro-breaks at 40 min intervals. Four main muscle areas were studied: the cervical extensors, the lumbar erector spinae, the upper trapezius/supraspinatus, and the wrist and finger extensors. It was determined ($p<0.05$) that micro-breaks had a positive effect on reducing discomfort in all areas studied during computer terminal work, particularly when breaks were taken at 20 min intervals. Finally, micro-breaks showed no evidence of a detrimental effect on worker productivity.

Village et al. (2005) worked on high injury rates in Intermediate Care (IC) facilities and the unclear factors related to these injuries. Their objectives of this exploratory sub-study, which was part of a large multi-faceted study in 8 IC facilities were to: (1) evaluate EMG measured over a full-shift in the back and shoulders of 32 care aides (CAs) as an indicator of peak and cumulative workload (n=4×8 facilities); investigate the relationship between EMG measures and injury indicators; and explore the relationship between EMG measures and other workload measurements. They converted lumbar EMG predicted cumulative spinal compression and ranged in CAs from 11.7 to 22.8 MN s with a mean of 16.4 MN s. Their results indicated that the average compression was significantly different during different periods of the day ($p<0.001$) with highest compression during pre-breakfast when CAs assist most with activities of daily living. Significant differences were found in average compression between low and high injury facilities for 3 of 5 periods of the day ($p<0.010$). Peak compressions exceeding 3400 N occurred for very little of the workday (e.g. 11.25 s during the 75 min period pre-breakfast). In their study the peak neck/shoulder muscle activity was low (99% APDF ranged from 8.33% to 28% MVC). They also indicated that peak and cumulative spinal compression were significantly correlated with lost-time and musculoskeletal injury rates as well as with total tasks observed in the CAs ($p<0.01$), perceived exertion was only correlated with peak compressions ($p<0.01$). Also they stated facilities with low injury rates provided significantly more CAs ($p<0.01$) to meet resident needs, and subsequently CAs performed fewer tasks, resulting in less peak and cumulative spinal loading over the day.

Menegaldo et al. (2006) showed a new method to estimate the muscle forces in musculoskeletal systems based on the inverse dynamics of a multi-body system associated optimal control. Their redundant actuator problem was solved by minimizing a time-integral cost function, augmented with a torque-tracking error function, and muscle dynamics is considered through differential constraints. Their method was compared to a previously implemented human posture control problem, solved using a Forward Dynamics Optimal Control approach and to classical static optimization, with two different objective functions. Their new method provided very similar muscle force patterns when compared to the forward dynamics solution, but the computational cost was much smaller and the numerical robustness is increased. Their results achieved suggested that this method was more accurate for the muscle force predictions when compared to static optimization, and can be used as a numerically 'cheap' alternative to the forward dynamics and optimal control in some applications.

Helland et al. (2008) investigated the effect of moving from single occupancy offices to a landscape environment. Thirty-four Visual Display Unit (VDU) operators reported significantly worsened condition of lighting and glare in addition to increased visual discomfort. Their results showed that for visual discomfort, the difference with 95% confidence interval was 10.7 (1.9–19.5) Visual Analog Scale (VAS) as group mean value. They indicated that the operators were glared from high luminance from the windows, when the Venetian blinds were not properly used. Moreover, according to their results glare was significantly correlated with visual discomfort, r_s=0.35 and both illuminance and luminance in the work area, and contrast reduction on the VDU screen were in line with recommendations from CIE for VDU work. Through a regression analysis, they showed that the visual discomfort explained 53% of the variance in the neck and shoulder pain. They found a marked drop in eye blink rate during VDU work when this was compared to "easy conversation" (VDU work, mean=9.7 blinks per minute; "easy conversation," mean=21.4 blinks per minute) for 12 randomly selected operators from the 34 participants. In their study, participants reported many of the organizational and psychosocial conditions and work factors worse when landscape office was compared to single occupancy office. It was indicated that these factors may have influenced the musculoskeletal pain. However, the pain level was still low at 6 years and not significantly different when compared with the start of the study period, except for a small but significant increase in shoulder pain. In their study, visual discomfort was clearly associated with pain in the neck and shoulder area.

11. Psychological Factors

Steingrímsdóttir et al. (2005) studied the relationship between musculoskeletal or psychological complaints and muscular responses to standardized cognitive and motor tasks. Their design examined (i) whether complaint severity predicts muscular responses during standardized tasks and (ii) whether the muscular responses predict changes in complaint severity over one year. They recorded musculoskeletal and psychological complaints by monthly reports the four months preceding and 12 months succeeding a work session in the laboratory; complaint-severity indices were computed from complaint-severity scores (intensity score × duration score). They also recorded surface electromyography (EMG) bilaterally from the upper trapezius, middle deltoid, and forearm extensor muscles in 45 post-office workers (30 women) during two identical task series. Between the series, they performed exhausting submaximal muscle contractions (25% of peak torque). In their adjusted regression models, no relations between musculoskeletal complaints the last four months and muscle activity during the task series were found. However, in their study psychological complaints in the last four months predicted higher muscle activity levels and a steeper rise in muscle activity in the muscles not engaged in motor task performance. Their results also showed that sleep disturbance was the strongest individual predictor of increased muscle responses. In contrast, they predicted psychological complaints the last four months lower EMG levels in the task-engaged muscle during the complex-choice-reaction-time tasks. Moreover, they stated that none of the muscle-activity responses to the standardized tasks predicted changes in severity of musculoskeletal or psychological complaints over the subsequent one-year period.

12. Effect of Interventions

It was shown that there was a US $17.8 return on investment for every dollar invested in an ergonomics intervention strategy. As a result of the redesign of an assembly line process, the worker compensation costs for work-related musculoskeletal disorders were reduced from $94,000 to $12,000 in a telecommunications organization. Between 1990 and 1994, ergonomics intervention saved $1.48 million in worker compensation costs for the same organization (Hendrick, 1996).

Mekhora et al. (2000) investigated the long-term effects of ergonomic intervention on neck and shoulder discomfort among computer users who have symptoms of tension neck syndrome, using simple materials and protocols. They conducted two pre-tests to determine subjects' level of discomfort before the planned intervention commenced. Discomfort evaluations (head, neck, shoulders, arms, and back) were conducted eight times within 6 months for both groups. The same patterns of decrease in the levels of discomfort of all body parts were present in both groups. They observed substantial variation in the level of discomfort over time for each body part in each subject after the intervention. However, the mean levels of discomfort ratings before and after receiving intervention were significantly different. They concluded that ergonomic intervention can help reduce the discomfort level of subjects with tension neck syndrome.

Lewis et al. (2002) assessed the effectiveness of an office ergonomics training program for VDT users in their study. They examined the worker compensation costs and injury rates for the VDT related musculoskeletal disorders before and after implementation of training at two company locations. The average cost per claim was considerably reduced from $15,141 in the pre-intervention period to $1553 in the post-intervention period. The average injury rate also reduced in the post (6.94 per 1000 employees) versus pre-intervention period (16.8 per 1000 employees).

Nevala-Puranen et al. (2003) compared the effects of two different intervention models for VDU work (E=redesign measures for the environment only, ET=redesign measures for both the environment and work techniques) on neck, shoulder and arm symptoms. They measured work posture, monitor viewing, muscular activity, and musculoskeletal pain for 20 participants before and after the 7-month intervention. Their results showed that there was a statistically significant difference between the groups for change in shoulder flexion ($p=0.0134$) and the muscular activity of right trapezius ($p=0.04109$) and right extensor carpi radialis ($p=0.0379$) in the pre- and post-intervention measurements. Additionally, the reduction of pain symptoms in the neck ($p=0.0073$), shoulders ($p=0.0071$) and elbows ($p=0.0490$) was greater in the ET group than in the E group.

Baldwin (2004) analyzed the problem of chronic disability associated with musculoskeletal disorders from an economic perspective, focusing on the small fraction cases with extraordinarily high costs. She reviewed the evidence on the costs of musculoskeletal disorders in general, and back pain in particular, identifying the sources of disproportionately high costs. Then, focusing on work-related back cases, she reviews the empirical evidence on workplace characteristics and economic incentives associated with long term disability and large productivity losses.

In their study, Bernaards et al. (2007) assessed the effectiveness of a single intervention targeting work style and a combined intervention targeting work style and physical activity on the recovery from neck and upper limb symptoms. They randomized computer workers with frequent or long-term neck and upper limb symptoms into the work style group (WS, $n = 152$), work style and physical activity group (WSPA, $n = 156$), or usual care group ($n = 158$). During the study the WS and WSPA group attended six group meetings. All meetings focused on behavioral change with regard to body posture, workplace adjustment, breaks and coping with high work demands (WS and WSPA group) and physical activity (WSPA group). They measured pain, disability at work, days with symptoms and months without symptoms at baseline and after 6 (T1) and 12 months (T2). They also assessed self-reported recovery at T1/T2. Both of their interventions were ineffective in improving recovery. Their work style intervention but not the combined intervention was effective in reducing all pain measures. They found that these effects were present in the neck/shoulder, not in the arm/wrist/hand. Furthermore, for the neck/shoulder, the work style intervention group also showed an increased recovery-rate. They observed total physical activity increased in all study groups but no differences between groups.

Lin and Chan (2007) studied the effect of ergonomic workstation design on musculoskeletal risk factors (MRFs) and musculoskeletal symptoms (MSSs) reduction among female semiconductor fabrication room (fab) worker. They conducted a prospective study to follow up 40 female fab workers over 3 months after intervention. The intervention program focused on reducing shoulder loadings for 20 female fab workers by redesigning nine workstations. They made simultaneous comparisons for the other 20 female fab workers using original workstations. They used one customized observation checklist and Nordic musculoskeletal questionnaire to evaluate workers' MRFs and MSSs, respectively. They found that one month after intervention, MRFs of awkward shoulder postures and repetitive motions and MSSs in shoulders for the intervention group were significantly lower than those for the control group. The lowering effects persisted for 3 months on awkward shoulder postures but lasted for only 1 month on repetitive motions and shoulder symptoms after intervention.

Escorpizo (2008) presented a *conceptual* model of work productivity—within the area of paid work and within the context of WMSD. He provided a discussion provided on the two components of work productivity, which are *perceived*and *observed* and between absenteeism and presenteeism as sub-components of work productivity. He stated that an accurate measurement of work productivity was crucial to initiating, evaluating, and monitoring work disability management like employee wellness and ergonomics programs, and clinical interventions in WMSD. He also presented a list of research agenda that can influence the ways we make use of *work productivity* as an outcome measure in capturing WMSD-associated socioeconomic burden and in evaluating WMSD management programs.

Musculoskeletal disorders (MSDs) affect much of the workforce and remain a major form of occupational ill health. With a view to improving the efficacy of interventions, this review examined preventative actions relating to these disorders. Denis et al. (2008) used a detailed analysis grid to classify the information contained in the 47 reviewed articles whose common aspect was to report actions carried out in the workplace that led to the implementation of changes to prevent MSDs. Their analysis identified and characterized three major categories of intervention processes in MSD prevention: the complete type (*n*=17), the shortened type (*n*=16), and the turnkey type (*n*=14). These three groups of intervention processes were differentiated by their approaches and their contexts of application. Their result was important differences in the changes implemented.

Robertson et al. (2009) undertook a large-scale field intervention study to examine the effects of office ergonomics training coupled with a highly adjustable chair on office workers' knowledge and musculoskeletal risks. They assigned office workers to one of three study groups: a group receiving the training and adjustable chair (*n*=96), a training-only group (*n*=63), and a control group (*n*=57). They created office ergonomics training program using an instructional systems design model and they administered a pre/post-training knowledge test to all those who attended the training. They observed body postures and workstation set-ups before and after the intervention. Their results indicated that perceived control over the physical work environment was higher for both intervention groups as compared to workers in the control group. Also, they observed a significant increase in overall ergonomic knowledge for the intervention groups. Their both intervention groups exhibited higher level behavioral translation and had lower musculoskeletal risk than the control group.

COMPUTER WORKSTATION ERGONOMICS CHECKLIST

	YES	NO
Lean back in chair to support your vertebrae	☐	☐
Elbows form a 90 degree angle while hanging at sides from the shoulders	☐	☐
Feet are comfortable on the floor in front of you	☐	☐
Your seat and your hands are centered on the keyboard	☐	☐
Sit symmetrically (not bending either sides)	☐	☐
The keyboard and the mouse are at the fingertips	☐	☐
The keyboard and the mouse are on the same level (side by side)	☐	☐
The screen is about an arm's length away from the eyes	☐	☐
The top of the monitor is at the eye level	☐	☐
Sufficient lightening available without glare from lights, windows, surfaces, and etc…	☐	☐
Neutral position of the wrist (straight from fingers to the elbow)	☐	☐
Neutral position of the head and the neck	☐	☐
Elbow/arm support provided for intensive/long durations	☐	☐
Leg support provided for intensive/long durations	☐	☐
Change sitting position at least every 15 minutes	☐	☐
Take active breaks (phone call, file paper, drink water, etc…) every 30 minutes	☐	☐
Take frequent microbreaks (while seated on your workstation)	☐	☐

REFERENCES

1. Aaras, A., Horgen, G., Bjorset, H. H., Ro, O., Thoresen, M., 1998. Musculoskeletal, visual and psychological stress in VDU operators before and after multidisciplinary ergonomic interventions. Applied Ergonomics 29 (5), 335-354.

2. Allread, W. G., 2000. An Investigation of the Relationship between Personality and Risk Factors for Musculoskeletal Disorders. Dissertation Abstracts International, vol. (2-B), 1019.

3. Amell, T. K., Kumar, S., 1999. Cumulative trauma disorders and keyboarding work. International Journal of Industrial Ergonomics 25, 69-78.

4. Aptel, M., Aublet-Cuvelier, A., Cnockaert, J. C., 2002. Work-related musculoskeletal disorders of the upper limb 69, 546-555.

5. Babski-Reeves, K. L., Crumtpon-Young, L. L, 2002. Comparisons of measures for quantifying repetition in predicting carpal tunnel syndrome. International Journal of Industrial Ergonomics 30(1), 1-6.

6. Babski-Reeves, K. L., Stanfield, J., Hughes, L., 2005. Assessment of video display workstation set up on risk factors associated with the development of low back and neck discomfort. International Journal of Industrial Ergonomics 35, 593-604.

7. Baker, N.A., Jacobs, K., Tickle-Degnen, L., 2003. The association between the meaning of working and musculoskeletal discomfort. International journal of Industrial Ergonomics 31 (4), 235-247.

8. Baker, N. A., Cham, R., Cidboy, E. H., Cook, J., Redfern, M. S., 2007. Kinematics of the fingers and hands during computer keyboard use. Clinical Biomechanics. Vol. 22 (1), 34-43.

9. Balcı, R., Aghazadeh, F., 2003. The effect of work-rest schedules and type of task on the discomfort and performance of VDT users. Ergonomics 46 (3), 455-465.

10. Baldwin, M. L., 2004. Reducing the costs of work-related musculoskeletal disorders: targeting strategies to chronic disability cases. Journal of Electromyography and Kinesiology 14, 33-41.

11. Baron, S., Hales, T., Hurrell, J., 1996. Evaluation of symptom surveys for occupational musculoskeletal disorders. American Journal of Industrial Medicine, 29 (6), 609–617.

12. Berkhout, A. L., Hendriksson-Larsen, K., Bongers, P., 2004. The effect of using a laptopstation compared to using a standard laptop PC on the cervical spine torque, perceived strain and productivity. Applied Ergonomics, 35 (2), 147-52.

13. Bernaards, C. M., Ariëns, G. A. M., Knol , D. L., Hildebrandt, V. H., 2007. The effectiveness of a work style intervention and a lifestyle physical activity intervention on the recovery from neck and upper limb symptoms in computer workers. Pain, Vol. 132 (1-2), 142-153.

14. Blatter, B. M., Bongers, P. M., 2002. Duration of computer use and mouse use in relation to musculoskeletal disorders of neck or upper limb. International Journal of Industrial Ergonomics 30, 295-306.

15. Bongers, P. M., de Winter, C. R., Kompier, M. A., Hildebrandt, V. H., 1993. Psychosocial Factors at Work and Musculoskeletal Disease. Scandinavian Journal of Work, Environment & Health, vol. 19 (5), 297-312.

16. Borghouts, J. A. J., Koes, B. W., Vondeling, H., Bouter, L. M., 1999. Cost of illness of neck pain in the Nedherlands in 1996. Pain 80, 629-636.

17. Broberg, E., 1996. *Anmälda* arbetssjukdomar i Norden 1990–1992 (Reported occupational diseases in the Nordic countries 1990–1992). The Nordic Council of Ministers, TemaNord, p. 545.

18. Buckle, P. W., Devereux J. J., 2002. The nature of work-related neck and upper limb musculoskeletal disorders. Applied Ergonomics 33, 207–217.

19. Carayon, P., Smith, M. J., Haims, M. C., 1999. Work Organization, Job Stress, and Work-Related Musculoskeletal Disorders. Human Factors 41 (4), 644-663.

20. Carey, E. J., Gallwey, T. J., 2002. Effects of wrist posture, pace and exertion on discomfort. International Journal of Industrial Ergonomics 29, 85-94.

21. Cham, R., Redfern, M.S., 2001. Effect of flooring on standing comfort and fatigue. Human Factors 43 (3), 381-391.

22. Chaparro, A., Bohan, M., Fernandez, J., Choi, S. D., Kattel, B., 1999. The impact of age on computer input device use: Psychophysical and physiological measures. International Journal of Industrial Ergonomics 24, 503-513.

23. Cook, C., Burgess-Limerick, R., Chang, S., 2000. The prevalence of neck and upper extremity musculoskeletal symptoms in computer mouse users. International Journal of Industrial Ergonomics 26 (3), 347-356.

24. Cook, C., Burgess-Limerick, R., 2004. The effect of forearm support on musculoskeletal discomfort during call centre work. Applied Ergonomics 35, 337-342.

25. Cook, C., Burgess-Limerick, R., Papalia, S., 2004. The effect of upper extremity on upper extremity posture and muscle activity during keyboard use. Applied Ergonomics 35, 285-292.

26. Cook, C., Burgess-Limerick, R., Papalia, S., 2004. The effect of wrist rests and forearm support during keyboard and mouse yse. International Journal of Industrial Ergonomics 33, 463-472.

27. Cooper, A., Straker, L., 1998. Mouse versus keyboard use: A comparison of shoulder muscle load. International Journal of Industrial Ergonomics 22, 351-357.

28. Coury, H. J. C. G., Porcatti, I. A.,Alem, M. E. R., Oishi, J., 2002. Influence of gender on work-related musculoskeletal disorders in repetitive tasks. International Journal of Industrial Ergonomics 29, 33-39.

29. David, G., Woods, V., Li, G., Buckle, P., 2008. The development of the Quick Exposure Check (QEC) for assessing exposure to risk factors for work-related musculoskeletal disorders. Applied Ergonomics, Vol. 39 (1), 57-69.

30. Denis, D., St-Vincent, M., Imbeau, D., Jetté, C., Nastasia, I., 2008. Intervention practices in musculoskeletal disorder prevention: A critical literature review. Applied Ergonomics, Vol. 39 (1), 1-14.

31. Dennerlein, J. T., Johnson, P. W., 2006. Different computer tasks affect the exposure of the upper extremity to biomechanical risk factors. Ergonomics 49 (1), 45-61.

32. Editorial, 2002. Muscular disorders in computer users: introduction. International Journal of Industrial Ergonomics 30, 203-210.

33. Erdil, M., Dickerson, O. B.. Cumulative Trauma Disorders: Prevention, Evaluation, and Treatment. John Wiley & Sons, 1996 (ISBN-10: 0442010745, ISBN-13: 9780442010744).

34. Escorpizo, Reuben. 2008. Understanding work productivity and its application to work-related musculoskeletal disorders. International Journal of Industrial Ergonomics, Vol. 38 (3-4), 291-297.

35. European Agency for Safety & Health at Work. Work-related Neck and Upper Limb Musculoskeletal Disorders (EU Agency Health & Safety Work). Commission of the European, December 30, 1999 (ISBN-10: 9282881741, ISBN-13: 978-9282881743).

36. Evans, O., Patterson, K., 2000. Predictors of neck and shoulder pain in non-secretarial computer users. International Journal of Industrial Ergonomics 26, 357-365.

37. Fagarasanu, M., Kumar, S., 2003. Carpal Tunnel Syndrome due to keyboarding and mouse tasks: a review. International Journal of Industrial Ergonomics 31 (2), 119-136.

38. Fernandez, J. E., Agarwal, R., Landwehr, H. R., Poonawala, M. F., Garcia, D. T., 1999. The effects of arm supports during light assembly and computer work tasks. International Journal of Industrial Ergonomics 24, 493-502.

39. Ferreira Jr., M., Sladiva, P. H. N., 2002. Computer-telephone interactive tasks: predictors of musculoskeletal disorders according to work analysis and workers' perception. Applied Ergonomics 33, 147-153.

40. Ferrigno, I. S. V., Cliquet Jr, A., Magna, L. A., Filho, A. Z., 2009. Electromyography of the Upper Limbs During Computer Work: A Comparison of 2 Wrist Orthoses in

Healthy Adults. Archives of Physical Medicine and Rehabilitation, Vol. 90 (7), 1152-1158.

41. Flodgren G., Heiden, M., Lyskov, E., Crenshaw, A. G., 2007. Characterization of a laboratory model of computer mouse use—Applications for studying risk factors for musculoskeletal disorders. Applied Ergonomics, Vol. 38 (2), 213-218.

42. Fogleman M., Lewis, R. J., 2002. Factors associated with self-reported musculoskeletal discomfort in video display terminal (VDT) users. International Journal of Industrial Ergonomics 29, 311-318.

43. Gerard, M. J., Armstrong, T. J., Rempel, D. A., 2002. The effects of work pace on within-participant and between-participant keying force, electromyography, and fatigue. Human Factors 44 (1), 51-61.

44. Goldenhar, L.M., Swanson, N.G., Hurrell, J.J. Jr., Ruder, A. & Deddens, J. Stressors and adverse health outcomes for female construction workers. Journal of Occupational Health Psychology, Vol 3(1) 1998, 19-32.

45. Grosch, J. and Murphy, L.R. Occupational Differences in Depression and Global Health: Results from a National Sample of U.S. Workers. Journal of Occupational and Environmental Medicine, Vol 40 1998, 153-164.

46. Hagberg, M., Silverstein, B. A., Wells, R. V., Smith, M. J., Hendrick, H. W., Carayon, P., Pérrusse, M., 1995. Work Related Musculoskeletal Disorders: A Reference for Prevention. Taylor&Francis, London.

47. Hair, J. F. Jr., Anderson, R. E., Tatham, R. L., Black, W. C. Multivariate Data Analysis: With Readings, Prentice Hall, February 1995, 4th edition.

48. Harvey, R., Peper, E., 1997. Surface electromyography and mouse use position. Ergonomics 40 (8), 781-789.

49. Helland, M., Horgen, G., Kvikstad, T. M., Garthus, T., Bruenech, J. R., Aarås, A., 2008. Musculoskeletal, visual and psychosocial stress in VDU operators after moving to an ergonomically designed office landscape. Applied Ergonomics, Vol. 39 (3), 284-295.

50. Helliwell, P., 1996. Diagnostic criteria for work-related upper limb disorders. Br. J. Rheumatorl 35, 1195-1196.

51. Hendrick, H. W., 1996. The ergonomics of economics is the economics of ergonomics. Ergonomics 8, 7-16.

52. Hudiburg, Richard A.; Pashaj, Irena; Wolfe, Raymond. Preliminary Investigation of Computer Stress and the Big Five Personality Factors. Psychological Reports, Vol 85(2) Oct 1999, 473-480.

53. Hudiburg, Richard A.; Necessary, James R. Coping with Computer-Stress. Journal of Educational Computing Research. Vol 15(2) 1996, 113-124. Baywood Publishing Co Inc.

54. Hudiburg, Richard A. Psychology of Computer Use: XXXIV. The Computer Hassles Scale: Subscales, Norms, and Reliability. Psychological Reports. Vol 77 (3, Pt 1) Dec 1995, 779-782.

55. Jensen, C., Finsen, L., Søgaard, K., Christensen, H., 2002. Musculoskeletal symptoms and duration of computer and mouse. International Journal of Industrial Ergonomics 30 (4-5), 265-275.

56. Jacobs, K., Johnson, P., Dennerlein, J., Peterson, D., Kaufman, J., Gold, J., Williams, S., Richmond, N., Karban, S., Firn, E., Ansong, E., Hudak, S., Tung, K., Hall, V., Pencina, K., Pencina, M., 2009. University students' notebook computer use. Applied Ergonomics, 404-409.

57. Jonai, H., Villanueva, M. B. G., Takata, A., Sotoyamam, M., Saito, S., 2002. Effects of the liquid crystal display tilt angle of a notebook computer on posture, muscle activities and somatic complaints. International Journal of Industrial Ergonomics 29, 219-229.

58. Karlqvist, L., Tornqvist, E. W., Magberg, M., Hagman, M., Toomingas, A., 2002. Self-reported working conditions of VDU operators and associations with musculoskeletal symptoms: a cross-sectional study focusing on gender differences. International Journal of Industrial Ergonomics 30, 277-294.

59. Klein, Jonathan T. TR#480: Computer Response to User Frustration. *MIT SM Thesis*, January 1999. (ftp://whitechapel.media.mit.edu/pub/tech-reports/TR-480.pdf)

60. Keir, P.J., Wells, R.P., 2002. The effect of typing posture on wrist extensor muscle loading. Human Factors 44(3), 392-403.

61. Korhan, Orhan. "Association of Emotions and Musculoskeletal Stress in Computer Users: An Occupational Risk Assessment Modelling". Lambert Academic Publishing, Germany 2010. ISBN: 978-3-8383-5525-2.

62. Korhan, O., Mackieh A. 2010. A Model for Occupational Injury Risk Assessment of Musculoskeletal Discomfort and Their Frequencies in Computer Users. Safety Science, Vol. 48 (7), 868-877.

63. Konz, S. A., Mital, A., 1990. Carpal tunnel syndrome. International Journal of Industrial Ergonomics 5 (2) 175-180.

64. Kothiyal, K., Kayis, B., 2001. Workplace layout for seated manual handling tasks: an electromyography study. International Journal of Industrial Ergonomics 27, 19-32.

65. Lee, D. L., McLoone, H., Dennerlein, J. T., 2008. Observed finger behaviour during computer mouse use. Applied Ergonomics, Vol. 39 (1), 107-113.

66. Lewis, R. J., Krawiec, M., Confer, E., Agopsowicz, D., Crandall, E., 2002. Musculoskeletal disorder worker compensation costs and injuries before and after an office ergonomics program. International Journal of Industrial Ergonomics 29, 95-99.

67. Liao, M. H., Drury, C. G., 2000. Posture, discomfort and performance in a VDT task. Ergonomics 43 (3), 345-359.

68. Lim, S.Y. & Murphy, L.R. Stress: Its impact on organizational effectiveness. In O. Baron Jr. & H.W. Hendrick (Eds.), Human factors in organizational design and management. Amsterdam, Netherlands: Elsevier Science B.V. (1996), pp 285-287.

69. Lin, R. T., Chan, C. C., 2007. Effectiveness of workstation design on reducing musculoskeletal risk factors and symptoms among semiconductor fabrication room workers. International Journal of Industrial Ergonomics, Vol. 37 (1), 35-42.

70. Marklin, R. W., Simoneau, G. G., Monroe, J. F., 1999. Wrist and forearm posture from typing on split and vertically inclined computer keyboards. Human Factors 41 (4), 559-569.

71. Marshall, M. M., Mozrall, J. R., Shealy, J. E., 1999. The effects of complex wrist and forearm posture on wrist range of motion. Human Factors 41 (2), 205-213.

72. Matias, A. C., Salvendy, G., Kuczek, T., 1998. Predictive models of carpal tunnel syndrome causation among VDT operators. Ergonomics 41, 213-226.

73. McBeth, J., Jones, K., 2007. Epidemiology of chronic musculoskeletal pain. Best Practice & Research Clinical Rheumatology. Vol. 21 (3), 403-425.

74. McLean, L., Tingley L., Scott, R. N., Rickards, J., 2002. Computer terminal work and the benefit of microbreaks. Applied Ergonomics 33, 1-8.

75. Mekhora, K., Liston, C. B., Nanthanvanij, S., Cole, J. H., 2000. The effect of ergonomic intervention on discomfort in computer users with tension neck syndrome. International Journal of Industrial Ergonomics 26, 367,-379.

76. Melin, Bo; Lundberg, Ulf. A Biopsychosocial Approach to Work-Stress and Musculoskeletal Disorders. *Journal of Psychophysiology*, Vol 11(3) 1997, 238-247.

77. Menegaldo, L. L., Fleury, A. T., Weber H. I., 2006. A 'cheap' optimal control approach to estimate muscle forces in musculoskeletal systems. Journal of Biomechanics, Vol. 39 (10), 1787-1795.

78. Menzel, Nancy N., 2007. Psychosocial Factors in Musculoskeletal Disorders. Critical Care Nursing Clinics of North America, Vol. 19 (2), 145-153.

79. Ming, Z., Zaproudina, N., 2003. Computer use related upper limb musculoskeletal (ComRULM) disorders. Pathophysiology 9, 155-160.

80. Muss, T., Hedge, A., 1999. Effects of a vertical split-keyboard on posture, comfort, and performance. Proceedings of the Human Factors and Ergonomics Society 43rd Annual Meeting, vol. 1, 496-500.

81. Muss, T., Barrero, M., 1999. Comparative study of two computer mouse designs. Cornell Human factors Laboratory Technical Report. /RP7992.

82. Nag, P. K., Pal, S., Nag, A., Vyas, H., 2009. Influence of arm and wrist support on forearm and back muscle activity in computer keyboard operation. Applied Ergonomics, Vol. 40 (2), 286-291.

83. Nevala-Puranen, N., Pakarinen, K., Louhevaara, V., 2003. Ergonomic intervention on neck, shoulder, and arm symptoms of newspaper employees in work with visual display units. International Journal of ındustrial Ergonomics 31, 1-10.

84. Østensvik, T., Veiersted, K. B., Nilsen, P., 2009. A method to quantify frequency and duration of sustained low-level muscle activity as a risk factor for musculoskeletal discomfort. Journal of Electromyography and Kinesiology, Vol. 19 (2), 283-294.

85. Panel on Musculoskeletal Disorders and the Workplace, 2001. Musculoskeletal disorders and the workplace: low back and upper extremities-Executive Summary. Theoretical Issues in Ergonomics Science 2 (2), 142-152.

86. Park, M. Y., Kim., J. Y., Shin, J. H., 2000. Ergonomic design and evaluation of a new VDT workstation chair with keyboard-mouse support. International Journal of Industrial Ergonomics 26, 537-548.

87. Peper, E., Wilson, V. S., Gibney, K. H., Huber, K., Harvey, R., Shumay, D.,M., 2003. The integration of electromyography (SEMG) at the workstation: assessment, treatment, and prevention of repetitive stain injury (RSI). Applied Psychophysiology and Biofeedback 28 (2), 167-182.

88. Press, S. J., Wilson, S., 1978. Choosing between Logistic Regression and Discriminant Ananlysis. Journal of American Statistical Association 73 (364), 699-705.

89. Punnett, L., Bergqvist, U., 1997. Visual Display Unit Work and Upper Extremity Musculoskeletal Disorders. A Review of Epidemiological Findings. National Institute for Working Life - Ergonomic Expert Committee Document No 1, 1997:16.

90. Punnett, L., Wegman, D. H., 2004. Work-related musculoskeletal disorders: the epidemiologic evidence and the debate. Journal of Electromyography and Kinesiology 14, 13-23.

91. Richter, J. M., Slijper, H. P., Over, E. A. B., Frens, M. A., 2008. Computer work duration and its dependence on the used pause definition. Applied Ergonoics, Vol. 39 (6), 772-778.

92. Robbins, M., Johnson, I.P. Cunliffe, C., 2009. Encouraging good posture in school children using computers. Clinical Chiropractic, Vol. 12 (1), 35-44.

93. Robertson, M., Amick, B. C. III, DeRango, K., Rooney, T., Bazzani, L., Harrist, R., Moore, A. (2009). The effects of an office ergonomics training and chair intervention on worker knowledge, behavior and musculoskeletal risk. Applied Ergonomics, Vol. 40 (1), 124-135.

94. Roe, C., Knardahl, S., 2002. Muscle activity and blood flux during standardized data-terminal work. International Journal of Industrial Ergonomics 30, 251-264.

95. Samani, A., Holtermann, A., Søgaard, K., Madeleine, P., 2009. Active pauses induce more variable electromyographic pattern of the trapezius muscle activity during computer work. Journal of Electromyography and Kinesiology, Vol. 19 (6), 430-437.

96. Sauter, S.L. & Hurrell, J.J., Jr. Origins, content, and direction. Professional Psychology: Research and Practice, *Occupational health psychology.* Vol 30(2) 1999, 117-122.

97. Seppaelae, Pentti. Experience of Stress, Musculoskeletal Discomfort, and Eyestrain in Computer-Based Office Work: A study in Municipal Workplaces. *International Journal of Human-Computer Interaction.* Vol 13(3) Sep 2001, 279-304.

98. Shuval, K., Donchin, M., 2005. Prevalence of upper extremity musculoskeletal symptoms and ergonomic risk factors at a High-Tech company in Israel. International Journal of Industrial Ergonomics 35, 569-581.

99. Simoneau, G.G., Marklin, R.W., Monroe, J. F., 1999. Wrist and forearm postures of users of conventional computer keyboards. Human Factors 41 (3), 413-424.

100. Simoneau, G.G., Marklin, R.W., 2001. Effect of computer keyboard slope and height on wrist extension angle. Human Factors 43 (2), 287-298.

101. Sommerich, C. M., Starr, H., Smith, C. A., Shivers, C., 2002. International Journal of Industrial Ergonomics 30, 7-31

102. Sprigg, C. A., Stride, C. B., Wall, T. D., Holman, D. J., Smith, P. R. , 2007 Work Characteristics, Musculoskeletal Disorders, and the Mediating Role of Psychological Strain: A Study of Call Center Employees. Journal of Applied Psychology, Vol. 92 (5), 1456-1466.

103. Steingrímsdóttir, Ó. A., Vøllestad, N. K., Knardahl, S., 2005. A prospective study of the relationship between musculoskeletal or psychological complaints and muscular responses to standardized cognitive and motor tasks in a working population. European Journal of Pain, Vol. 9 (3), 311-324.

104. Straker, L., Jones, K. J., Miller, J., 1997. A comparison of the postures assumed when using laptop computers and desktop computers. Applied Ergonomics 28 (4), 263-268.

105. Straker, L., Mekroha, K., 2000. An evaluation of visual display unit placement by electromyography, posture, discomfort and preference. International Journal of Industrial Ergonomics 26, 389-398.

106. Straker, L., Burgess-Limerick, R., Pollock, C. Murray K. Netto, K. Coleman, J., Skoss, R., 2008. The impact of computer display height and desk design on 3D posture during information technology work by young adults. Journal of Electromyography and Kinesiology, Vol. 18 (2), 336-349.

107. Straker, L., Burgess-Limerick, R., Pollock, C., Maslen, B., 2009. The effect of forearm support on children's head, neck and upper limb posture and muscle activity during computer use. Journal of Electromyography and Kinesiology, Vol. 19 (5), 965-974.

108. Suh, Hyunsuk. Risk Perception in Work Organization Musculoskeletal Discomfort and Stress. *Dissertation Abstracts International*, Vol 61 (5-B) Dec 2000, 2702.

109. Szabo, R. M., 1998. Carpal tunnel syndrome as a repetitive motion disorder. Clinical Orthopaedics 351, 78-89.

110. Szeto, G. P. Y., Straker, L. M., O'Sullivan, P. B., 2005. The effects of speed and force of keyboard operation on neck-shoulder muscle activities in symptomatic and asymptomatic office workers. International Journal of Industrial Ergonomics 35, 429-444.

111. Szeto, G. P. Y., Straker, L. M., O'Sullivan, P. B., 2005. The effects of typing speed and force on motor control in symptomatic and asymptomatic office workers. International Journal of Industrial Ergonomics 35 (9), 779-795.

112. Szeto, G. P.Y., Sham, K. S.W., 2008. The effects of angled positions of computer display screen on muscle activities of the neck–shoulder stabilizers. International Journal of Industrial Ergonomics, Vol. 38 (1), 9-17.

113. Szeto, G. P. Y., Straker, L. M., O'Sullivan· P. B., 2009. Neck–shoulder muscle activity in general and task-specific resting postures of symptomatic computer users with chronic neck pain. Manual Therapy, Vol. 14 (3), 338-345.

114. Tayyari, F., Emanuel, J. T., 1993. Carpal tunnel syndrome: An ergonomics approach to its prevention. International Journal of Industrial Ergonomics 11 (3), 173-179.

115. Tepper, M., Vollenbroek-Hutten M. M. R., Hermens, H. J., Baten, C. T. M., 2003. The effect of an ergonomic computer device on muscle activity of the upper trapezius muscle during typing. Applied Ergonomics 34, 125-130.

116. Thorn, S., Søgaard, K., Kallenberg, L. A. C., Sandsjö, L. , Sjøgaard, G., Hermens, H. J., Kadefors, R., Forsman, M., 2007. Trapezius muscle rest time during standardised computer work – A comparison of female computer users with and without self-reported neck/shoulder complaints. Journal of Electromyography and Kinesiology, Vol. 17 (4), 420-427.

117. Tittiranonda, P., Rempel, D., Armstrong, T., Burastero, S., 1999. Effect of four computer keyboards in computer users with upper extremity musculoskeletal disorders. American Journal of Industrial Medicine 35, 647-661.

118. Toomingas, A., 1998. Methods for evaluating work-related musculoskeletal neck and upper-extremity disorders in epidemiological studies. Arbetslivinstitutet (National Institute for Working Life). Arbete Och Halsa Vetenskaplig Skriftserie 6.

119. Vergera, M., Page, A., 2002. Relationship between comfort and back posture and mobility in sitting posture. Applied Ergonomics 33, 1-8.

120. Village, J., Frazer, M., Cohen, M., Leyland, A., Park, I., Yassi A. (2005). Electromyography as a measure of peak and cumulative workload in intermediate care and its relationship to musculoskeletal injury: An exploratory ergonomic study. Applied Ergonomics, Vol. 36 (5), 609-618.

121. Wadman, C., Kjellberg A., 2007. The role of the affective stress response as a mediator for the effect of psychosocial risk factors on musculoskeletal complaints—Part 2: Hospital workers. International Journal of Industrial Ergonomics, Vol. 37 (5), 395-403.

122. Weigl, M., Cieza, A., Cantista, P., Stucki, G., 2007. Physical disability due to musculoskeletal conditions. Best Practice & Research Clinical Rheumatology, Vol. 21 (1), 167-190.

123. Westgaard, R. H., 2000. Work-related musculoskeletal complaints: some ergonomics challenges upon the start of a new century. Applied Ergonomics 31, 569-580.

124. Won, E. J., Johnson, P. W., Punnett, L., Dennerlein, J. T., 2009. Upper extremity biomechanics in computer tasks differ by gender. Journal of Electromyography and Kinesiology, Vol. 19 (3), 428-436.

125. Wu, J. Z. An, K. N., Cutlip, R. G., Krajnak, K., Welcome, D., Dong, R. G., 2008. Analysis of musculoskeletal loading in an index finger during tapping. Journal of Biomechanics, Vol. 41 (3), 668-676.

LaVergne, TN USA
08 October 2010
200192LV00002B/6/P